Healthy Eating, Healthy Weight for Kids and Teens

Jodie Shield, MEd, RD,
and Mary Catherine Mullen, MS, RD

D0054516

 Eat Right Press

EAT RIGHT PRESS
Published by Academy of Nutrition and Dietetics
Diana Faulhaber, Publisher
Laura Pelehach, Acquisitions and Development Manager
Elizabeth Nishiura, Production Manager

The views expressed in this publication are those of the authors and do not necessarily reflect policies and/or official positions of the Academy of Nutrition and
Dietetics. Mention of product names in this publication does not constitute en-
dorsement by the authors or the Academy of Nutrition and Dietetics. The Academy of Nutrition and Dietetics disclaims responsibility for the application of the
information contained herein.

For more information on the Academy of Nutrition and Dietetics,
go to *www.eatright.org*

10 9 8 7 6 5 4 3 2 1

ISBN 978-0-9837255-0-3

Contents

Acknowledgments

I would like to dedicate this book to my beautiful mother, Marilyn Ann Collins, July 19, 1937–June 7, 2011, and to my healthy family (Jim, Michael, JJ, and Jennifer) and the summer of 2010—keep the faith!

Jodie Shield, MEd, RD

Thanks to my family for their patience, support, and love. Thanks to all my co-workers at Rush University Medical Center, who work so hard to get the message to families to be healthy. Most importantly, thanks to Jodie for her determination to write this book. Your countless hours and dedication made this book become a reality.

Mary Mullen, MS, RD

The authors and the Academy of Nutrition and Dietetics also gratefully acknowledge the contributions of the peer reviewers for this book: Katie Brown, EdD, RD, Nancy Copperman, MS, RD, CDN, and Denise Sofka, MPH, RD.

Introduction

Are you concerned about your child's weight? You're not alone. *All* parents want their kids to be a healthy weight. However, as the media reminds us every day, we are in the midst of an obesity epidemic. Over the past twenty years, kids' weights have skyrocketed. Generally speaking, children today weigh about 10 pounds more than kids did 30 years ago, and one out of three American kids is currently overweight or obese.

As parents, we love our children no matter what their size or shape—they are not statistics! On the other hand, helping them achieve and maintain a healthy weight is more important than ever. Did you know the following facts?

- Being obese after the age of six is a strong predictor of adult obesity.
- Seventy percent of obese teens go on to become obese adults.
- Twenty-five percent of obese adults were overweight as children, and more severe obesity in adults is associated with having been overweight before age eight.

Why Weight Matters

Being overweight is a risky business. In adults, overweight and obesity are linked to six of the 10 leading causes of illness and death in the United

States: heart disease, cancer, stroke, chronic lower respiratory diseases, diabetes, and kidney diseases. Because overweight children have a greater probability of becoming obese adults, our kids could be headed for a future of health problems. In fact, for many kids, the future is now. Overweight and obese youths are beginning to experience weight-related health issues sooner rather than later. That is to say, kids are developing medical conditions that used to only affect adults. Here are a few you should know about:

- *Type 2 diabetes:* Type 2 diabetes is associated with overweight and obesity, and it used to be rare in kids. Before 1994, the incidence of type 2 diabetes in children and teens was less than 5 percent. Since that time, it has risen dramatically to between 30 and 50 percent. Early onset of type 2 diabetes puts kids at a greater risk of developing cardiovascular diseases (such as high blood pressure and high cholesterol) and kidney disease.
- *Hypertension:* High blood pressure among kids is also on the rise. Approximately 13 percent of overweight or obese children have elevated systolic blood pressure (the upper number) and approximately 9 percent have elevated diastolic blood pressure (the lower number). Untreated, hypertension can lead to heart attacks and strokes.
- *Hyperlipidemia:* Hyperlipidemia, or high levels of fat in the blood, is one of the most common obesity-related medical conditions in children and teens. Overweight children (especially boys) are more likely to have elevated levels of total cholesterol and LDL cholesterol (the bad type). This puts them at greater risk for serious heart disease.
- *Early puberty:* Obese children tend to begin puberty earlier than healthy weight children. This may predispose them to physical and psychological changes that they are intellectually not ready to handle. Also, kids who enter puberty early tend to not grow as tall as their peers who enter puberty at a later age.
- *Polycystic ovary syndrome (PCOS):* Obese teenage girls are at increased risk for PCOS, an imbalance in a girl's hormone levels that leads to irregular or missed periods.

- *Sleep disorders:* Sleep disorders such as sleep apnea occur in about 17 percent of obese children and teens. Sleep apnea is when people stop breathing for short periods of time while sleeping. It is a serious problem, and kids who have sleep apnea often perform poorly in school.
- *Asthma:* Asthma is a lung disease in which the airways become blocked or narrowed and results in breathing difficulty. Overweight children, particularly boys, seem to be at a greater risk of developing asthma, and being overweight seems to aggravate the symptoms in kids who already have asthma. Obese children with asthma tend to use more medicine, wheeze more, and visit the emergency room more often than their peers with asthma who are not obese.
- *Orthopedic problems:* Overweight and obese kids often develop orthopedic or bone abnormalities. These problems seem to be a direct result of carrying too much weight and overloading the growing skeletal frame, particularly in areas that involve the growth plates, such as knees, ankles, and hips.
- *Psychosocial problems:* Some of the most devastating problems that affect overweight and obese kids are psychological in nature. Their weight often interferes with their ability to relate to other family members and peers, and may lead to depression. They may find it challenging to play outside at recess, keep up with friends at the park, or wear the latest styles. Other kids at school may also tease them. Researchers have found that, compared to healthy weight peers, severely obese children and teens are about five times more likely to report having a lower quality of life. Overweight youth often have lower self-esteem and tend to feel lonely, sad, and nervous. They are also more likely to smoke and consume alcohol and may be socially isolated. Weight issues also can cause body dissatisfaction, which may place kids, particularly girls, at risk for eating disorders.

This list is not meant to scare you. However, it is important for parents to know the very serious health problems that some overweight and obese kids currently face.

Help Is on the Way!

If your child is trying to reach a healthy weight, this book is for you. (It can even help if your child is already a healthy weight.) You'll learn how your child's weight fits into the big picture. You'll gain tips for raising a healthy eater in a fattening world, and you'll explore eight successful *Healthy Eating, Healthy Weight* strategies recommended by the world's largest organization of food and nutrition professionals, the Academy of Nutrition and Dietetics (*www.eatright.org;* formerly the American Dietetic Association). Backed by years of research, these eight strategies can help your child or teen reach and maintain a healthier weight. Studies have also found that each of these strategies may be essential to preventing unhealthy weight gain in kids currently at a healthy weight, as the strategies promote healthy eating habits that will last a lifetime.

My coauthor, Mary, and I are both registered dietitians (RDs) and members of the Academy of Nutrition and Dietetics. For the past 25 years, we have been in the trenches helping families learn how to eat healthier and achieve a healthy weight. Over the past several years, we've noticed that more and more families have been coming to us for help, particularly about their child's or teen's weight. While there are many resources to help adults with their weight, we really couldn't find much for kids. So, we felt it would be helpful to write this book. *Healthy Eating, Healthy Weight for Kids and Teens* is the perfect blend of science and real-world experience. As moms, Mary and I collectively have seven kids between the ages of 12 and 23 years. We are right there with you as parents—we know firsthand how challenging it can be to get a preschooler to nibble on broccoli and enjoy eating cauliflower; convince a grade-schooler to spend more time playing basketball instead of video or computer games; help a tween to understand the word "mobile" means move your body, not make a cellphone call; persuade a teenager to drink milk instead of soft drinks and to slow down on fast food; and arrange for the family (even Dad!) to sit down and eat dinner together on a regular basis.

The causes of the obesity epidemic are likely a combination of genetic, behavioral, and environmental factors. We can't change our genetic make-up (yet), but families *can* improve their behavior and change how they interact with their environment. Therefore, *Healthy Eating, Healthy Weight for*

Kids and Teens is a book for the whole family, and it emphasizes personal responsibility. The research is very clear on this issue: parents need to be responsible for selecting and offering healthy foods; kids need to be responsible for how much of food they choose to eat. However, for many families, the line dividing these responsibilities has been crossed—by both parties. Luckily, there are solutions. As parents, we are our children's first and best teachers and their most influential role models. It would be fair to say we are their heroes. This book will empower you with the knowledge and tools you need to help your kids achieve a healthier weight in the fattening world in which they live and play.

How to Use This Book

Healthy Eating, Healthy Weight for Kids and Teens is not a book that you need to read linearly, from cover to cover. We recommend that you start by reading Chapters 1 and 2 because they lay the groundwork for the rest of the book, first by helping you identify whether your child or teen is a healthy weight (Chapter 1) and then by outlining the eight *Healthy Eating, Healthy Weight* strategies covered in this book and helping you choose which strategy to try first (Chapter 2). Chapter 2 also provides a couple of essential tools—the family goal contract and a tracking form—that enable your family to commit to goals related to a *Healthy Eating, Healthy Weight* strategy and measure your progress toward those goals.

After you explore these first chapters, you make the call where to go next! Each of the following eight chapters (Chapters 3 through 10) covers a particular *Healthy Eating, Healthy Weight* strategy, and you can read them in any order, as best suits your family's needs. You'll find tips, tools, and possible goals to lead your family to success. These chapters are framed by the stories of other families facing weight challenges and feature "Weigh In" quotes from kids and parents who are tackling the specific strategy. We hope these personal voices help you remember that you are not alone (note: we've changed names and fictionalized some scenarios). Finally, Chapter 11 concludes the book with three weeks' worth of sample menus to help you plan *Healthy Eating, Healthy Weight* family meals and snacks. This chapter also offers more than 40 kid-tested-and-approved healthy recipes.

Next Steps

Healthy Eating, Healthy Weight for Kids and Teens can help everyone in the family (kids *and* parents) learn how to eat healthier and reach a healthier weight. This book embraces the Academy of Nutrition and Dietetics philosophy that "all foods can fit" into a healthy lifestyle, and that the "family approach" is the best way to help kids achieve and maintain a healthy weight. However, no book can ever take the place of medical advice. If you suspect that your son or daughter is overweight or obese, we highly recommend that you follow up with your pediatrician. Some kids might need more help or may not be able to lose weight without medical supervision. Your pediatrician will be able to perform additional laboratory tests to accurately assess your child's health. In addition, he or she can recommend an RD to help you fine tune your family's eating and physical activity habits. Even if your son or daughter is at a healthy weight (*see* Chapter 2), an annual physical exam is still a good idea.

Stay In Touch

We encourage you to read *Healthy Eating, Healthy Weight for Kids and Teens* and use it over and over. Share the information in this book with grandparents, caregivers, teachers, and everyone who feeds your child. Bring the book with you to your child's annual health check up and discuss it with your pediatrician. Also, be sure to talk to your child or teen about the information you learn in this book. Throughout the chapters, we've listed a variety of interactive Web sites where you and your child can learn even more.

Last, but not least, we hope you will stay in touch! Join the conversation by visiting our blog *(www.HealthyEatingForFamilies.com)* or interacting with us on Facebook and Twitter *(@eating_healthy)*. We will keep you updated on *Healthy Eating, Healthy Weight for Kids and Teens*.

—Jodie Shield, MEd, RD, and Mary Catherine Mullen, MS, RD

1

What Is a Healthy Weight?

■ *Ten-year-old Peter usually looks forward to playing youth football, but this season he wants to quit. At registration, the coaches told Peter he weighed too much; he would have to move up a level to play with the junior high boys. Peter asked his mom, Lucy, "Am I fat?" Sensing her son's embarrassment and disappointment, she replied, "No! You're just big." But deep down, she wasn't sure. Folks kept commenting on how "big" Peter had gotten. At Peter's fifth grade physical, his pediatrician confirmed Lucy's fear: her son was too heavy.* ■

When you were growing up, how many times did your grandma or a close family friend hug you and say, "You're getting *so* big!"? Odds are you heard this plenty of times. Were you or your parents offended? Probably not. At one time, "big" was code for mature or grown up. Fast-forward to today. How do you feel if somebody says your son or daughter is getting "so big"? Like Peter and his parents, you might not take the comment as a compliment, especially if it comes from a pediatrician. This chapter will help you determine whether your child's or teen's weight is healthy.

How Does Your Child's Weight Measure Up?

When adults gain weight, there are all kinds of signs. We can no longer squeeze into our favorite jeans or we loosen our belts a few notches. And, of course, the bathroom scale never lies. But it's much trickier to tell whether a child or teen is overweight. Since kids are still growing, they need to gain weight *and* they are supposed to outgrow their clothes. Also, since kids grow and develop at different ages, you can't simply look at them and conclude they are overweight (*see* What Is Normal Growth?). The best way to determine whether your child's weight is healthy is for you to measure and keep track of his or her *body mass index (BMI)*. That's what pediatricians do, and you can do it, too.

WHAT IS NORMAL GROWTH?

Kids grow at different times and rates, and there is a wide range of "normal" growth patterns. Here are some *average* growth statistics to help you gauge your youngster's progress:

- *Preschool:* Between the ages of two and five years, the average child grows about 2½ inches and gains four to five pounds each year.
- *Middle childhood:* During the grade school years, kids grow at a steady pace. Each year they get about two inches taller and gain anywhere from 5 to 10 pounds.
- *Preadolescence:* During preadolescence, most children, especially girls, gain weight primarily in the form of body fat. Preadolescent weight gain often occurs between the ages of 9 and 11 in girls and 10 and 12 in boys. This weight gain is normal and necessary to help them prepare for the rapid and intense growth spurt that will occur in adolescence.
- *Adolescent growth spurt:* In this growth spurt, many kids lose their "extra" body fat and grow into their weight. During this time, adolescents achieve the final 15 to 20 percent of their adult height. The age range in which kids reach this growth spurt varies greatly.

BMI: Know Your Child's Number

For years, pediatricians have used height and weight measurements to compare your child's growth to other boys and girls the same age. Now they have another tool: BMI, a number calculated from your child's height and weight that can be used to estimate body fat. BMI does not measure body fat directly, but many studies have shown that it is a reliable indicator of body fatness and disease risk for most kids (*see* Introduction). Plus, it's an inexpensive and simple method for determining whether a child's or teen's weight is healthy. In fact, it's so simple, you can calculate your own son's or daughter's BMI with an ordinary calculator or by using an online tool. Just keep in mind that to calculate BMI accurately, you must start by obtaining an accurate height and weight (*see* Scaling New Heights).

SCALING NEW HEIGHTS

What is the most accurate way to measure your kid's height and weight? Here are the methods that the Centers for Disease Control and Prevention (CDC) recommend.

To measure weight:

1. Use a digital scale. Avoid using bathroom scales that are spring-loaded. Place the scale on firm flooring (such as tile or wood) rather than carpet.
2. Have the child or teen remove shoes and heavy clothing, such as sweaters.
3. Have the child or teen stand with both feet in the center of the scale.
4. Record the weight to the nearest decimal fraction (for example, 55.5 pounds or 25.1 kilograms).

To measure height:

1. Remove the child's shoes, bulky clothing, and hair ornaments, and unbraid hair that interferes with the measurement.
2. Take the height measurement on flooring that is not carpeted and against a flat surface such as a wall with no molding.

(continued)

SCALING NEW HEIGHTS *(continued)*

3. Have the child stand with feet flat, together, and against the wall. Make sure legs are straight, arms are at sides, and shoulders are level.

4. Make sure the child is looking straight ahead and that the line of sight is parallel with the floor.

5. Take the measurement while the child stands with head, shoulders, buttocks, and heels touching the wall. Depending on the overall body shape of the child, all points may not touch the wall.

6. Use a flat headpiece to form a right angle with the wall and lower the headpiece until it firmly touches the crown of the head.

7. Make sure the measurer's eyes are at the same level as the headpiece.

8. Lightly mark where the bottom of the headpiece meets the wall. Then, use a metal measuring tape to measure from the base on the floor to the marked measurement on the wall to get the height measurement.

9. Accurately record the height to the nearest ⅛th inch or 0.1 centimeter.

Adapted from Centers for Disease Control and Prevention. About BMI for Children and Teens. *www.cdc.gov/healthyweight/assessing/bmi/childrens _bmi/measuring_children.html.*

How to Calculate BMI

You don't need to be a math whiz to calculate BMI. Just grab your calculator and use one of the two basic BMI formulas. It doesn't matter which formula you use since they both end up with the same BMI—so you make the call.

Formula 1:

BMI = Weight (pounds) ÷ Height (inches) ÷ Height (inches) × 703

Formula 2:

BMI = Weight (kilograms) ÷ Height (centimeters)

÷ Height (centimeters) × 10,000

Note: After you have done the math, round off the BMI to the nearest whole number.

Let's calculate BMI for Peter, the boy profiled at the start of this chapter. If Peter weighs 129 pounds (59 kilograms) and is 63 inches (160 centimeters) tall, his BMI is 23.

Formula 1: BMI = 129 ÷ 63 ÷ 63 × 703 = 23

Formula 2: BMI = 59 ÷ 160 ÷ 160 × 10,000 = 23

What is your kid's BMI? Calculate your child's or teen's BMI using either of the formulas (or use the online method described on page 9). Write the BMI here: _____

Interpreting BMI

When BMI is used to evaluate weight in an adult, the BMI number alone is sufficient to place the individual in a weight category (underweight, normal, overweight, or obese). However, we can't use an adult BMI chart for kids because their body fatness changes as they grow. Also, girls and boys differ in body fatness, especially as they mature, so we need to use gender-specific criteria for evaluating BMI in kids.

To address these differences between adults and kids and between girls and boys, health care professionals use *BMI-for-age percentile* growth charts to interpret BMI in boys and girls ages 2 to 20 years. These graphs list ages along the y axis (vertically) and BMI along the x axis (horizontally), and show curves for different BMI percentiles. To use a BMI growth chart, you plot (mark) the point on the graph where your child's age and BMI cross, and then take note

Kids Weigh In: Extra Credit

I got extra credit in math for teaching my class how to calculate their BMI.

—MADDIE, AGE 11

of either the percentile curve the point lands on or the curves on either side of this point. The percentiles of those curves become the key to understanding whether the BMI is in a healthy range. You can access a chart online *(www.cdc.gov/growthcharts);* we also show you an example of the chart for boys on page 8.

How do you interpret your child's or teen's BMI percentile? Based on pediatric body fat research, medical experts have come up with the following weight categories for children and teens:

- **Underweight**: BMI is less than the 5th percentile.
- **Healthy weight**: BMI is between the 5th and 84th percentiles.
- **Overweight**: BMI is between the 85th and 94th percentiles.
- **Obese**: BMI is equal to or greater than the 95th percentile.

When we plot the BMI for 10-year-old Peter, we find that his BMI of 23 puts him above the 95th percentile for his age, which means he is in the obese category. **What is your kid's BMI percentile category?** Write it down here: _____.

Note: It's important to point out that "overweight" and "obese" are medical terms and should not be used in front of kids. It's best to talk to your child or teen about being a healthy weight (*see* Weight: A Heavy Topic for Kids).

WEIGHT: A HEAVY TOPIC FOR KIDS

Heavy kids often have problems with their body image and self-esteem. Before talking with your child or teen about weight, carefully review the following recommendations—each is backed up with scientific research:

- *Talk about "healthy weight."* Always emphasize the importance of being a healthy weight when talking with your child or teen. Categories such as overweight and obese are medical terms to discuss privately with your kid's pediatrician and registered dietitian.

WEIGHT: A HEAVY TOPIC FOR KIDS *(continued)*

- *Stay positive.* Parents who criticize their sons and daughters about their weight are more likely to have overweight kids. Overweight kids probably know better than anyone else that they have a weight problem. What they need most is support, understanding, and encouragement.
- *Give kids a hug.* Tell your kids how special you think they are and how much you love them. Kids' feelings about themselves are often based on how they think their parents feel about them.
- *Focus on your family.* Instead of singling out one particular child, make healthy eating and physical activity a family affair.
- *All food can fit.* Studies have found that restricting foods is associated with overweight in children. Instead of forbidding certain foods, help your child learn how to eat and enjoy all food in smaller portions.

Tracking BMI over Time

A single BMI calculation does not tell your child's whole weight story. As kids grow, their body fat changes, which means their BMI will change, too. That is why it's important to track BMI over time. To illustrate this point, let's compare the BMI of 23 (Peter's BMI) for boys at two different ages. At age 10, Peter's BMI is above the 95th percentile for his age and in the obese category. However, a 15-year-old boy with a BMI of 23 would be between the 5th and 85th percentiles and in the healthy weight category (*see* the sample growth chart).

BMI: A Word of Caution

BMI is the gold standard for *screening* potential weight problems—it cannot be used to make a final diagnosis. For example, if your child or teen is very athletic and muscular, his or her BMI may be high because of extra muscle mass, not body fat (muscle weighs more than fat). If your son's or

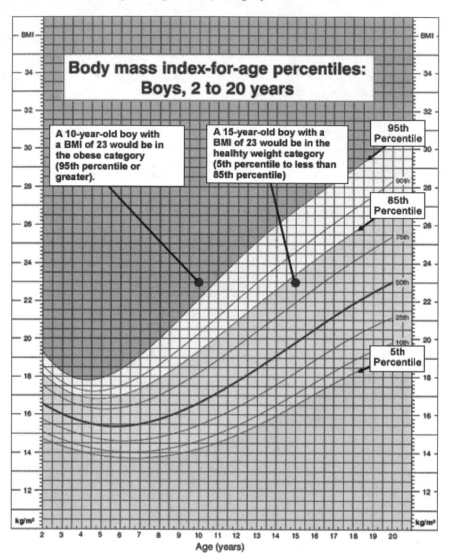

Body Mass Index (BMI) Growth Chart Comparing a BMI of 23
for Boys Ages 10 and 15

HOW TO FIND A REGISTERED DIETITIAN

A registered dietitian (RD) is a food and nutrition expert who has met tough academic and professional requirements which includes completing a minimum of a four-year bachelor's degree and an accredited, supervised practice program (an internship). Some RDs are also certified in specialized areas of practice such as weight management or diabetes education.

To find an RD in your area, ask your child's pediatrician for a recommendation or use the Academy of Nutrition and Dietetics *Find a Registered Dietitian* service. Just go to the Academy's Web site *(www.eatright.org)* and click *Find a Registered Dietitian* at the top of the Home page. Fill in the requested information, and a list of highly qualified RDs will be at your fingertips.

daughter's BMI falls in the overweight or obese category, consider this to be a *warning sign,* not an absolute diagnosis. Before you take drastic measures such as putting your child on a diet, talk with your child's pediatrician or a registered dietitian (*see* How to Find a Registered Dietitian).

Calculating Your Child's BMI Online

Many BMI calculator tools are available online. One of the best is the BMI Percentile Calculator for Child and Teen, which is available for free from the CDC. To access it, go to: *http://apps.nccd.cdc.gov /dnpabmi* (since technology is ever changing, we also have a link to the calculator on our Web site: *www.HealthyEatingForFamilies.com*). To use the calculator, fill in your son's or daughter's birth date, height, and weight along with the current date. The program will automatically calculate the BMI. It also

Parents Weigh In: Adult BMI

After finding out my son's BMI, I was curious to know my own. I used the Adult BMI calculator on the CDC Web site *(www.cdc.gov)*. Turns out, I'm overweight!
—EIGHT-YEAR-OLD JIMMY'S DAD

offers feedback on how to interpret the number and lets you to track your child's BMI over time.

Healthy Eating, Healthy Weight—You're in Control

■ *After speaking privately to Peter's pediatrician, his parents understood that his BMI of 23 put him in the obese category. Peter's growth history showed that his BMI had always been on the lower end of overweight before jumping dramatically to this level. His mom, Lucy, went back to working full time a year ago, and Peter admitted that he snacked on chips, candy, and soda pop after school and through the evening. The pediatrician recommended a treatment approach that would help Peter safely reach a healthy weight while he was growing. The family went to see an RD, who worked with them to make specific lifestyle changes. Lucy learned how to plan healthier meals and snacks for Peter, and he agreed to switch from soda to water. Since everyone was concerned about Peter playing football with older kids, he signed up to play soccer with kids his own age instead. Peter made excellent progress. By the next football season, his BMI was back to where it used to be and the entire family was eating healthier. ■*

Congratulations! You have just taken the first major step in helping your child or teen achieve a healthy weight. Now you know how to:

- Calculate BMI and use online calculators.
- Use BMI percentiles to identify whether your child or teen may be healthy weight, overweight, or obese.
- Determine whether your child's or teen's current or future health may be at risk because of his or her weight.

Your next step is to read Chapter 2. It will give you the tools you need to choose a winning strategy for helping your child or teen achieve a healthy weight.

2

Which Weigh to Go? Healthy Eating, Healthy Weight Strategies for Kids and Teens

■ *Ever since she was cut from the basketball team, 15-year-old freshman Cassandra has gained several pounds. She has also resorted to hiding a stash of candy bars and chips under her bed since her mom declared these foods off limits. Cassandra is tired of her mom's nagging. Just because her mom is always on the latest diet, Cassandra doesn't see why she has to be on one, too. "I think I look fine!," she screeches at her mom.*

Cassandra used an online body mass index (BMI) calculator and learned that her BMI was at the 80th percentile for her age, which falls in the healthy weight range. She shared this finding with her mom, who seemed happy but still had concerns. Cassandra used to get so much exercise when she played basketball, but now she typically hangs out with her friends, eats fast food, and sends texts all day on her cellphone. Her mom worries that Cassandra will not be able to stay at a healthy weight if she continues this behavior. ■

As parents, we need to make healthy eating and physical activity a priority because they're two of the most important investments we can make for our child's or teen's future health. In Chapter 1, you learned how to calculate and interpret your son's or daughter's BMI. Like Cassandra and her mom, you're probably wondering—now what? If your child is overweight, should she lose a few pounds? If your teen's weight is healthy, how can he keep it that way? This chapter offers the latest recommendations for helping kids achieve and maintain a healthy weight. It will also identify eight *Healthy Eating, Healthy Weight* strategies and help you choose which strategies to pursue immediately with your child or teen.

Experts Weigh In on Kids and Weight Loss

Until recently, only one way to help overweight kids was recommended. Pediatricians and registered dietitians (RDs) agreed: never put children on weight-loss diets; instead, help families make healthy lifestyle changes and let the kids grow into their weight. For many kids, this approach, which is called *weight maintenance,* still works. However, there has recently been a lot of research on kids and weight, and weight loss *is* now recommended for some overweight kids to help them reach a healthy weight. Furthermore, kids who are obese or experiencing health problems such as high blood pressure or type 2 diabetes should lose weight under the supervision of their pediatrician and RD. For some obese kids with serious health complications, very low–calorie diets, medications, or even surgery might be treatment options—but only if they are working with a highly qualified medical team that specializes in obesity. In 2007 an Expert Committee made up of 15 major health organizations, released new science-based recommendations and strategies to help kids achieve and maintain a healthy weight. The recommendations are tailored for three age groups (2 to 5 years, 6 to 11 years, and 12 to 18 years) and broken down according to BMI percentiles. Keep in mind that these recommendations are meant to be *goals* that you and your child can strive to reach together, ideally with the help of an RD.

**Parents Weigh In:
Healthy Eating
Family-Style**

I am a pediatric nurse at a children's hospital in Chicago. Any child with a BMI above the 95th percentile is automatically referred to an RD. I've noticed when the whole family is involved in making changes, the child's weight improves.

—PATTY, RN

Healthy Weight Goals for Children Ages Two to Five Years

For children between the ages of two and five years, the following are the Healthy Weight goals recommended by the Expert Committee:

- **BMI between 5th and 84th percentiles (healthy weight)**: Keep BMI in the healthy weight range through healthy eating and physical activity.
- **BMI between 85th and 94th percentiles (overweight)**: Through healthy eating and physical activity, either slow down weight gain or try to maintain the child's current weight until BMI is less than the 85th percentile.
- **95th percentile or higher (obese)**: Through healthy eating, physical activity, *and* the help of an RD, maintain the child's current weight until the BMI is less than the 85th percentile. If the health care team recommends weight loss, it should not exceed one pound per month.

Healthy Weight Goals for Children Ages 6 to 11 Years

The following are the Expert Committee's Healthy Weight goals for children between the ages of 6 and 11 years:

- **BMI between 5th and 84th percentiles (healthy weight)**: Keep BMI in the healthy weight range through healthy eating and daily physical activity.
- **BMI between 85th and 94th percentiles (overweight)**: Through healthy eating and daily physical activity, either slow down weight gain or try to maintain the child's current weight until BMI is less than the 85th percentile.
- **BMI between 95th and 99th percentiles (obese)**: Either maintain the child's current weight until BMI is less than the 85th percentile or help the child lose about one pound per month with healthy eating, daily physical activity, *and* the help of an RD.
- **BMI above the 99th percentile (obese)**: Try to help the child lose no more than two pounds a week with the help of an RD and

other health professionals who have experience working with obese children.

Healthy Weight Goals Teens Ages 12 to 18 Years

The Expert Committee recommended the following Healthy Weight goals for teens:

- **BMI between 5th and 84th percentiles (healthy weight)**: Keep BMI in the healthy weight range through healthy eating and daily physical activity.
- **BMI between 85th and 94th percentiles (overweight)**: Through healthy eating and daily physical activity, either slow down weight gain or try to maintain the teen's current weight until BMI is less than the 85th percentile.
- **BMI between 95th and 99th percentiles (obese)**: Through healthy eating, daily physical activity, *and* the help of an RD, try to help the teen lose about two pounds a week until BMI is less than the 85th percentile.
- **BMI above the 99th percentile (obese)**: Try to help the teen lose no more than two pounds a week with the help of an RD and other health professionals who have experience working with obese teens.

Applying the Healthy Weight Goals

Let's see how the Healthy Weight goals apply to Cassandra, the teen profiled at the beginning of this chapter. As a teen whose BMI is at the 80th percentile (within the healthy weight range), her Healthy Weight goal should be to maintain her weight with healthy eating and daily physical activity.

What is your kid's Healthy Weight goal? Using your child's or teen's age and BMI percentile, scan through the Healthy Weight goals to find out what the experts recommend. Write the goal down here: _____

_____

_____

Healthy Eating, Healthy Weight: Show Me the Strategies!

You now know your son's or daughter's Healthy Weight goal. But what can you do to achieve it? While there are a variety of ways to help kids reach and maintain a healthy weight, all the advice can be boiled down into eight *Healthy Eating, Healthy Weight* strategies. We've listed them in no particular order of importance—because each and every one is important! When you're done building each strategy into your family's lifestyle, the end result will be healthy eating and healthy weight.

1. **Strategy #1**: Eat with a plan! Enjoy delicious family meals and snacks that are balanced and healthy.
2. **Strategy #2**: Turn off the tube and move! Reduce all screen time to less than two hours a day *and* be physically active 60 minutes or more a day.
3. **Strategy #3**: Pop the soda habit! Limit sugar-sweetened beverages (such as soda, sport drinks, and punch) to one serving or less a day.

> ### Kids Weigh In: Diets Don't Work
>
> I don't think diets work. My mom is always on a diet, but she always looks the same to me.
> —JOHNNY, AGE 12

4. **Strategy #4**: Practice portion control! Cut food and beverage portions down to the sizes recommended in MyPlate.
5. **Strategy #5**: Fill up on fruits and veggies! Eat plenty of servings of fruits and vegetables every day.
6. **Strategy #6**: Slow down the fast food! Limit fast food to less than once a week.
7. **Strategy #7**: Sound the alarm! Eat breakfast every morning.
8. **Strategy #8**: Come together! Eat family meals at least five times a week.

Where to Begin

Now that you've identified your child's or teen's Healthy Weight goals and reviewed the possible strategies, you're ready to step up to the healthy plate and help your child or teen—or the whole family—achieve a healthy weight. We've come up with a quiz to help you choose which strategy to work on first. Each of the eight *Healthy Eating, Healthy Weight* strategies has its own chapter. After your family masters one strategy, move on to another. Just remember to be patient. Changing eating and physical activity behaviors is hard work, and it takes time (*see* How to Make or Break a Habit on page 18). Remember also to be a good role model. Research shows that children and teens really do listen to their parents and follow their lead. If you eat well, move more, and spend less time in front of the TV or computer, your kids will, too. You are their *Healthy Eating, Healthy Weight* hero!

Healthy Eating, Healthy Weight—You're In Control

■ *Even though Cassandra's BMI was in the healthy weight range, she and her mom talked with her pediatrician, who recommended that they work with an RD named Eileen. Eileen went over the fundamentals of healthy eating with Cassandra and her mom and taught Cassandra how to make healthier choices when she ate fast food with her friends. Eileen also helped the family sort through some emotional issues. Cassandra admitted that she felt stressed starting high school and missed playing basketball, and she decided to join a local youth basketball league. Cassandra's mom agreed to be more supportive, stop making comments about Cassandra's weight, and let Cassandra have a say in the types of snack food they stocked in their kitchen.* ■

On your mark, get set, go! In this chapter, you learned:

- How to identify your child's or teen's weight management goals based on BMI.
- The eight *Healthy Eating, Healthy Weight* strategies that can help kids reach and maintain a healthier weight.
- Which of the eight *Healthy Eating, Healthy Weight* strategies may work best for your child and family.

HEALTHY EATING, HEALTHY WEIGHT FOR KIDS AND TEENS QUIZ

Take a few minutes to answer the following Yes or No questions. Choose "No" when you're not sure about your answer. If you answer "No," consider reading the recommended chapter for help with the related *Healthy Eating, Healthy Weight* strategy.

My child or teen . . .	Your answer	If you answered "No," read . . .
Eats regularly scheduled meals and snacks that are balanced and healthy *most of the time.*	Yes No	Chapter 3
Is physically active *60 minutes or more a day.*	Yes No	Chapter 4
Limits screen time (TV, computers, video games) to *less than 2 hours a day.*	Yes No	Chapter 4
Drinks sugar-sweetened beverages (soda, sport drinks, and punch) *less than once a* day.	Yes No	Chapter 5
Eats the serving sizes recommended in MyPlate (www.ChooseMyPlate.gov) most of the time.	Yes No	Chapter 6
Eats *at least five servings* of fruits and vegetables *every day.*	Yes No	Chapter 7
Eats fast food *no more than one time a week.*	Yes No	Chapter 8
Eats breakfast *every day.*	Yes No	Chapter 9
Eats family dinners *at least five or six times a week.*	Yes No	Chapter 10

HOW TO MAKE OR BREAK A HABIT

Habits are behaviors that we perform automatically—without think-ing—because we have done them so many times before. It takes time to form new, healthier habits. As a rule-of-thumb, people need about three weeks to establish a new behavior pattern and about three months to make it a habit. The exact time frame will vary, depending upon a person's motivation and the habit. For example, drinking a cup of water every morning is an easier habit to establish compared to doing 100 sit-ups before breakfast.

   Here are some tips for making healthy eating and physical activ-ity a habit for your child or teen:

* *Repetition is key.* Just as you learned multiplication tables by go-ing over them repeatedly, we learn healthy habits through daily repetition.
* *Practice!* Encourage your child to regularly practice the behavior at the same time and place. For example, if you want a kid to eat more fruit, offer her an apple every day for an afterschool snack.
* *Set the pace early.* Help your child follow through consistently with the new behavior, especially at the beginning. Your child can form a habit if he skips a day, but it will take longer to develop.

Which chapter are you going to read next? We suggest you start with whichever chapter covers the strategy you think will be most helpful for your child or teen. Each chapter offers tips and resources to help you suc-ceed and provides guidance on how to choose specific goals and achieve them.

   As you work your way through a strategy, involve the entire family in the process of setting goals and meeting them (*see* Goal Setting Tips). One technique that really works is to write a family contract to commit to work-ing on your goals and then record your progress in a simple tracking form (at the end of this chapter we've provided samples for you to use as models).

   For example, your family could set a goal to eat three meals every day (*see* Chapter 3). Write that goal down on your family goal contract. Then mark off every day that you meet it using your tracking card. You don't have to be perfect. If you hit the goal most of the time, that's great! Another goal could be to take an after-dinner walk as a family three or four times a week (*see* Chapter 4). Again, write the goal down and then keep track of the days you walked. Review your goals every week until you feel you have made lasting changes that promote a *Healthy Eating, Healthy Weight* lifestyle. When you have mastered one or two goals, move on to another one.

GOAL SETTING TIPS

- *Start as a family*. Sit down and come up with goals together. That way, everyone can take ownership and cooperate.
- *Set no more than three goals at a time*. If you try to make too many changes at once, your family will be overwhelmed.
- *Make each goal specific*. "Exercise more" is a great idea, but it is not specific. "Take family walks four times a week" is much more concrete.
- *Be realistic*. For example, the goal should fit your family's budget, schedule, and cooking skills. If a goal is complicated, costs a lot, or eliminates everyone's favorite foods, then your family is unlikely to stick with it.
- *Identify obstacles*. For example, you may have to ask grandma to stop bringing over a big batch of cookies every Sunday. Instead, maybe she could bring a fruit salad or just enough cookies for everyone to have one or two as a special treat.
- *Know that your family can do it*. Use the information and resources in this book to help your family stay positive and focused.
- *Forgive your lapses and celebrate successes*. Your family doesn't have to be perfect. If you miss a few days, relax. Get back on track as soon as you can. Remember, changing habits take time. When your family reaches a goal, reward yourselves with nonfood prizes, such as a trip to the movies or park.

SAMPLE FAMILY GOAL CONTRACT

Gather your family together to write and sign a contract listing the goals you plan to work on in the next week or two.

We the _____ family will work toward the following goal(s) over the next one or two weeks:

_____

_____

_____

When we have successfully made these a habit, we will reward ourselves with _____

_____

_____

_____

Signed:

_____

_____

_____

Adapted from Kosharek SM. *If Your Child Is Overweight: A Guide for Parents*. 3rd ed. Chicago, IL: American Dietetic Association; 2006.

SAMPLE TRACKING RECORD

Studies show that we do better when we keep track of our progress. Use the following tracking record to keep score of your family's healthy eating and physical activity goals each week. Check the box if you meet the goal that day. At the end of the week, gather your family together and discuss your progress. You'll be surprised at how keeping score helps you stay motivated!

My Goals

Name: _____

Date: _____ **Week:** _____

My Healthy Eating Goals	Sun	Mon	Tues	Wed	Thurs	Fri	Sat
My Physical Activity Goals	Sun	Mon	Tues	Wed	Thurs	Fri	Sat

Adapted from the Eat Hard, Play Smart Tracking Card published on the U.S. Department of Agriculture Food and Nutrition Service. Eat Smart, Play Hard, Healthy Lifestyle Web site.

www.fns.usda.gov/eatsmartplayhardhealthylifestyle/KeepScore/TrackingCard.pdf.

3

Healthy Eating, Healthy Weight Strategy #1: Eat with a Plan!

■ *Single mom Elizabeth Jackson has three kids—13-year-old Anthony, 8-year-old Kendra, and 4-year-old Keeshawn. Elizabeth works full time, while Keeshawn stays with his grandmother and the older kids attend school and an afterschool program run by the youth center. Elizabeth works long hours, and Gramma usually lets Keeshawn snack and watch TV until his mom can pick him up. Exhausted from her job and family commitments, Elizabeth tends to order pizza for dinner or grabs fast food like fried chicken or tacos for the family on her way home from work. Her weekends are jam-packed, too—laundry, errands, driving Kendra to dance class and Anthony to the mall to meet friends. Keeshawn tags along, feasting on bags of chips and sipping juice drinks. When the kids had their check-ups, the pediatrician told Elizabeth that the older kids' weights were healthy, but Keeshawn was too heavy for his age. To help him reach a healthy weight, and keep the older kids' weight in a healthy range, the pediatrician recommended that the whole family try* Healthy Eating, Healthy Weight Strategy #1: Eat with a plan! Enjoy delicious family meals and snacks that are balanced and healthy. ■

If your family is like the Jackson family—busy and pulled in a dozen different directions—then you know that eating well can be a challenge.

But the research is clear: for kids to be a healthy weight and healthier over-all, they need to eat balanced meals and snacks that are healthy—that is, light on foods with added sugar and solid fat while emphasizing foods that provide short-changed nutrients such as fiber, potassium, calcium, and vitamin D. This chapter will teach you how to create a customized daily food plan that is balanced, healthy, and easy for everyone in the family (kids *and* adults) to follow. Your family's daily food plan will include breakfast, lunch, dinner, and snacks. There will be no need to cook special meals. Everyone can eat the same foods, just in different amounts. You'll also find recommendations for online tools and Web sites to help everyone put healthy eating into action.

What Does Healthy Eating Look Like?

For your child or teen to be a healthy weight, everyone in the family needs to have a seat at the table and participate. Healthy eating should be a way of life for everyone, not just certain family members. Essentially, healthy eating for a healthy weight can be boiled down to the following:

- Eating the right *kinds* of foods—foods with maximum amounts of healthy nutrients and minimal amounts of added sugar and solid fat.
- Eating the right *amounts* of these foods, with choices from each of the five food groups—in other words, meals that are planned and balanced.

When kids eat the right types and amounts of food, they achieve a healthy weight and get the right mix of nutrients to nurture their growing bodies. However, most kids don't eat enough fruits and vegetables, whole grains, and dairy foods. Instead, they are drinking soda pop and eating foods with added sugar and solid fat, like doughnuts, cookies, candy, chips, and French fries. In fact, about 30 percent of the calories that kids get each day come from these types of foods, which provide extra calories without many vitamins and minerals. Desserts are a top-five calorie source for kids from ages 2 to 18. For teens ages 14 to 18, soda, pizza, and desserts are the top three sources of calories! In addition to eating poorly, kids fall short when it comes to physical activity and exercise, too. They seem to have traded in their gym shoes for TV remotes (*see* Chapter 4). As a result, many kids are gaining too much weight—they're overfed but undernourished.

That's the troubling news. The good news is that *you* have the power to establish healthier eating habits for your family. Read on for help with planning meals and snacks that balanced, healthy, and delicious.

Serving Up Healthy Eating—What's on Your Plate?

In 2011 the U.S. government introduced MyPlate, a new and improved icon for healthy eating. Like the Food Pyramid that it replaces, MyPlate is based on the Dietary Guidelines for Americans (*see* Key Messages of the 2010 Dietary Guidelines for Americans). However, MyPlate is much easier to use than the Food Pyramid ever was. All you have to do is glance at My-Plate and you'll get an instant snapshot of the role that each of the five food groups should play in healthy eating. For starters, vegetables and fruits are very important and should fill half the plate. Grains should take up the next largest section of the plate. The remaining plate space is reserved for protein foods (like lean meat and beans). Finally, off to the right, you'll notice a dairy circle as a reminder to include some calcium-rich foods, such as milk or yogurt.

Although the MyPlate icon can quickly remind you of what healthy eating looks like, the symbol cannot communicate how much or what types of food to eat. No worries. MyPlate also has a Web site *(www .ChooseMyPlate.gov)* where you can learn a great deal about healthy eating for a healthy weight. For example, click any of the food groups for information on recommended serving sizes, specific nutrients in various foods, and their unique health benefits. You'll also find all kinds of healthy eating tips and interactive tools (*see* MyPlate Tools and Tips on page 26). But before you check out the MyPlate Web site, let's explore each of the food groups.

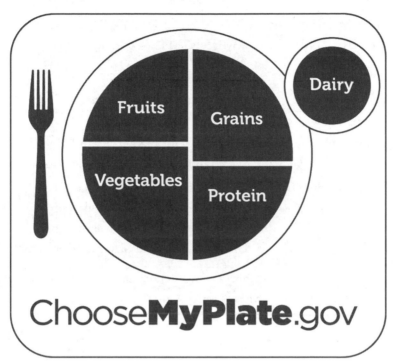

MyPlate Icon

KEY MESSAGES OF THE 2010 DIETARY GUIDELINES FOR AMERICANS

Every five years, the U.S. Department of Agriculture and the U.S. Department of Health and Human Services jointly publish the Dietary Guidelines for Americans *(www.dietaryguidelines.gov)*. Based on a nongovernmental panel's expert review of research related to eating, physical activity, and health, the 2010 Dietary Guidelines broke new ground by focusing directly on two of today's most important dietary issues: weight management and nutrient-dense foods. That is to say, the current Dietary Guidelines focus on healthy eating for a healthy weight. The chart highlights the three themes emphasized in the Dietary Guidelines, all of which have been incorporated into our eight *Healthy Eating, Healthy Weight* strategies:

(continued)

KEY MESSAGES OF THE 2010 DIETARY GUIDELINES FOR AMERICANS *(continued)*

Theme	Action Steps
Balancing calories	• Enjoy your food, but eat less.
	• Avoid oversized portions.
Foods to increase	• Make half your plate fruits and vegetables.
	• Switch to fat-free or low-fat (1%) milk.
Foods to reduce	• Compare sodium in foods like soup, bread, and frozen meals and choose the foods with lower numbers.
	• Drink water instead of sugary drinks.

Adapted from U.S. Department of Agriculture and U.S. Department of Health and Human Services. Dietary Guidelines for Americans, 2010. *www.dietaryguidelines.gov.*

MYPLATE TIPS AND TOOLS

The MyPlate Web site *(www.ChooseMyPlate.gov)* provides fun and interactive online materials that adults and kids can use to help eat healthy for a healthy weight, such as:

- *MyPlate Food Planner:* This tool lets you plan a menu and see how it will fit each family member's personal MyPlate daily food plan.
- *MyFood-a-pedia:* Not sure what food group pizza is in? How many calories are in a chocolate chip cookie? What's a healthier choice—a beef taco or chicken taco? MyFood-a-pedia provides instant access to all kinds of food information, such as food groups, calories, and comparisons. It can help you plan and evaluate MyPlate daily food plans quickly and accurately.

MYPLATE TIPS AND TOOLS *(continued)*

- *MyPlate Food Tracker:* An online food and activity diary, MyPlate Food Tracker can help anyone interested in healthy eating and a healthy weight. It gives immediate feedback on food and physical activity choices based on your child's or teen's specific MyPlate daily food plan. Teens particularly like this tool because it helps them better understand energy balance (calories eaten, calories burned) and healthy eating.

Touring the Food Groups

Your food group tour is about to begin. Each stop offers an overview of how a particular food group can help your child or teen eat healthy for a healthy weight. In each section, we'll cover the key nutrients, health benefits, and recommended serving sizes. You'll also find two types of food lists:

- *Go for It foods:* These are the foods kids should eat *every day* because they are rich in healthy nutrients. (A word of caution for parents of young children. Some foods, even healthy ones, can be hard for preschoolers to chew. If you have a preschooler, *see* Preschooler Choking Hazards on page 28.)
- *Take It Easy foods:* These foods have added sugar, solid fat, or both. Kids should cut way back on these foods because they offer too many calories and can lead to an unhealthy weight. If kids eat these foods, they should eat them only occasionally, in very limited portions, and only after eating all of their *Go for It* foods.

Let the tour begin!

PRESCHOOLER CHOKING HAZARDS

Preschoolers have a tough time trying to chew and swallow because they lack a full set of teeth. Some foods might even cause them to choke. These foods tend to be round and about the size of a nickel, which happens to be about the size of a young child's throat. Avoid serving these foods or be sure to cut them into tiny pieces (no larger than one-half inch).

Carrot sticks or baby carrots	Popcorn
Cherry or grape tomatoes	Raisins
Chewing gum	Seeds
Hard candy	Snack chips
Hot dogs or sausages	Whole grapes
Nuts	

Grains

Key Nutrients in Grains

Grains provide carbohydrate—the body's main energy source—which helps kids get up and go. Grains are also important sources of many other nutrients, including several B vitamins (thiamin, riboflavin, niacin, and folate) and minerals (iron, magnesium, and selenium). *Whole* grains are good sources of dietary fiber, a nutrient that most kids (and adults) do not get enough of. Fiber can help reduce blood cholesterol levels and may lower heart disease risk. Fiber also helps eliminate constipation and may play a role in weight control by helping to curb kids' appetites.

What Counts as a Serving?

A one-ounce serving from the grain group is equal to one slice of bread; one cup of ready-to-eat cereal; or one-half cup of cooked rice, cooked pasta, or cooked cereal.

How Many Servings Do Kids Need Each Day?

The number of grain servings that your child or teen needs will depend on his or her daily calorie needs (*see* Appendixes A and B). On the MyPlate Web site *(www.ChooseMyPlate.gov)*, check the Grains column on your son or daughter's MyPlate daily food plan to find the recommended number of servings listed in ounces.

Go For It *Grains: Make Half Your Grains Whole*

When choosing grain foods, read food labels to make sure they are enriched (*see* Enriched versus Fortified: What's the Difference?). Also, for healthy eating and a healthy weight, at least *half* of everyone's daily grain choices should be whole grains:

- *Whole grains* are the whole grain kernel with the bran, germ, and endosperm intact.
- *Refined grains* started out as whole grains, but they are processed to give them a finer texture and longer shelf life. During this process, the bran and germ are removed, which also removes dietary fiber, iron, and many B vitamins. Most refined grains are enriched with all of these missing nutrients except dietary fiber.

ENRICHED VERSUS FORTIFIED: WHAT'S THE DIFFERENCE?

If a food has been *enriched,* nutrients lost during the milling process are added back. Many breads, flours, and rice are enriched with B vitamins and iron. If a food has been *fortified,* nutrients that were never there originally are added to enhance the nutritional profile of the food and often to promote health. Some foods that are fortified include iodized salt (iodine is added to salt), milk and many yogurts (fortified with vitamins A and D), and calcium-fortified fruit juices.

Keep in mind that some foods are made from a mixture of whole grains and refined grains. Check the ingredients list and choose foods that have "whole grain" or "whole wheat" listed as one of the first ingredients (*see* Chapters 6 and 9). For more tips on helping your family eat more whole grains, *see* Kid-Friendly Whole Grain Tips.

EXAMPLES OF *GO FOR IT* GRAINS

Whole Grains

- Brown rice
- Buckwheat
- Bulgur (cracked wheat)
- Oatmeal (regular or instant but without added sugar)
- Popcorn (plain)
- Whole grain ready-to-eat breakfast cereals: whole wheat cereal flakes,* whole grain toasted oats,* whole grain shredded wheat*

- Whole grain barley
- Whole grain cornmeal
- Whole rye
- Whole wheat bread*
- Whole wheat crackers*
- Whole wheat pasta
- Whole wheat sandwich buns and rolls*
- Whole wheat pita*
- Whole wheat tortillas
- Wild rice
- "White" whole grain bread*

Refined Grains

- Corn tortillas
- Couscous
- Flour tortillas
- Grits
- Noodles and pasta (spaghetti, macaroni, etc.)

- Pitas*
- White bread*
- White sandwich buns and rolls*
- White rice

Note: Foods marked with an asterisk (*) may contain a small amount of added sugar.

KID-FRIENDLY WHOLE GRAIN TIPS

Here are a few pointers to help you make half your kid's daily grain choices whole grains:

- *Bulk up breakfast.* Start the day with a bowl of hot oatmeal or whole grain cereal with sliced banana and fat-free (skim) milk. Top a whole grain waffle or pancake with fat-free blueberry yogurt instead of syrup. Wrap scrambled eggs in a whole wheat tortilla for a quick breakfast burrito

- *Serve whole wheat sandwiches.* Turn an ordinary turkey or peanut butter sandwich into an extraordinary one by using whole grain breads. There are so many tasty whole wheat options, such as whole wheat pita pockets, English muffins, and mini-bagels. Stores even offer "white" whole grain bread now.

- *Use your noodle.* Make your favorite pasta dish with whole wheat noodles, such as angel hair, linguini, macaroni, corkscrew, or even whole wheat egg noodles. Whole wheat pasta tends to be a little chewier, so kids may need to get use to the taste. Start by using a mix of half whole wheat and half refined grain pastas.

- *Pump up pizza, soups, and stews.* Make or order pizza with a whole grain crust. Toss whole grains into soups and stews. Try adding barley to vegetable soup or bulgur to beef stew

- *Go wild with rice.* Skip the mashed potatoes and serve wild rice as your starch. Use brown rice instead of white in your favorite stir-fry or casserole recipe. If you're in a hurry, pick up a quick-cooking or instant brown rice—they're whole grain, too.

- *Bake and switch.* When a recipe calls for white flour, try replacing up to half of the flour with whole grain flour. If you want a lighter texture and color, try using white whole wheat flour.

- *Swap snacks.* Try a whole grain snack chip such as baked whole-grain tortilla chips. Or cook up some popcorn and top it off with a dash of salt-free seasoning or, for added flavor, a sprinkle of low-fat parmesan cheese.

- *Ask when you eat out.* Many restaurants now offer whole wheat bread and pasta with meals. So go ahead and ask if you can have it your whole-grain way.

Take It Easy *Grains*

Many foods in the Grain group have added sugar and solid fat, some much more than others. The *Take It Easy* foods we've listed are very high in calories compared to relative amount of healthy nutrients they provide. For healthy eating and a healthy weight, make sure your child or teen eats these foods only occasionally, in very limited portions, and only after eating all of his or her *Go for It* foods.

EXAMPLES OF *TAKE IT EASY* GRAINS

- Biscuits
- Cakes
- Cookies
- Cornbread
- Crackers
- Crisps and cobblers
- Croissants
- Doughnuts
- Granola bars
- Muffins
- Pastries and pies
- Sweetened breakfast cereals
- Sweet rolls

Vegetables

Key Nutrients in Vegetables

Eat your vegetables—they're good for you! That's what our parents always told us, and we need to share this wisdom with our kids, too. Vegetables are a nutritional powerhouse. They are low in calories but offer so many nutrients, including potassium, folate (folic acid), and vitamins A, E, and C. Vegetables also contain hunger-fighting dietary fiber as well as phytonutrients, which help prevent diseases such as cancer and heart disease (*see* Chapter 7).

What Counts as a Serving?

A one-cup serving of vegetables is equal to one cup of raw or cooked vegetables or vegetable juice or two cups of raw leafy greens.

How Many Servings Do Kids Need Each Day?

The recommended number of daily vegetable servings depends on a child's or teen's daily calorie needs. To find out how many servings of vegetables (in cups) your child or teen should eat, check the Vegetables column on his or her MyPlate daily food plan *(www.ChooseMyPlate.gov)* or see Appendixes A and B of this book.

Go For It *Vegetables: Vary Your Veggies*

When kids are hungry, always encourage them to eat more vegetables! Most vegetables are naturally low in fat; none have cholesterol; and they provide very few calories (unless prepared with added fats or other high-calorie ingredients—see the *Take It Easy* section below). Any fresh, frozen, canned, or dried/dehydrated vegetable counts as a member of the Vegetable group. One hundred percent vegetable juice also counts, but the whole vegetable offers more fiber than the juice. Vegetables may be whole, cut up, or mashed. They can also be raw or cooked.

Certain subcategories of vegetables offer different nutrients than other vegetable subcategories. Therefore, it's important to eat a wide variety of vegetables. To help your family with this goal, the *Go for It* chart (page 34) divides vegetables into five subcategories based on their similar nutrient content (for more information, *see* Chapter 7).

Take It Easy *Vegetables*

There are very few vegetables that kids should avoid (*see* page 35). However, preparing vegetables with butter or cream sauces adds solid fat, cholesterol, and calories. Deep-frying also adds solid fat and lots of extra calories. For healthy eating and a healthy weight, make sure your child or teen eats the *Take It Easy* types of vegetables only occasionally, in very limited portions, and only after eating all of his or her *Go for It* foods.

EXAMPLES OF *GO FOR IT* VEGETABLES

Dark-Green Vegetables

- Bok choy
- Broccoli
- Collard greens
- Kale
- Romaine lettuce
- Spinach
- Turnip greens

Red and Orange Vegetables

- Acorn squash
- Butternut squash
- Carrots
- Pumpkin
- Sweet potatoes

Beans and Peas

- Black beans
- Black-eyed peas
- Garbanzo beans (chickpeas)
- Kidney beans
- Lentils
- Navy beans
- Pinto beans
- Soybeans
- Split peas
- White beans

Starchy Vegetables

- Corn
- Green peas
- Lima beans (green)
- Potatoes

Other Vegetables

- Artichokes
- Asparagus
- Bean sprouts
- Beets
- Brussels sprouts
- Cabbage
- Cauliflower
- Celery
- Cucumbers
- Eggplant
- Green beans
- Green or red peppers
- Iceberg (head) lettuce
- Mushrooms
- Okra
- Onions
- Parsnips
- Zucchini

EXAMPLES OF *TAKE IT EASY* VEGETABLES

- Avocados (naturally high in fat)
- French fries
- Onion rings
- Potato chips

Fruits

Key Nutrients in Fruits

Fruits are so important for healthy eating and a healthy weight. Most are naturally low in fat, sodium, and calories, and none have cholesterol. Fruits are excellent sources of many nutrients including potassium, vitamin C, folate (folic acid), and phytonutrients. Fruits also provide dietary fiber which may help kids feel full and curtail overeating. *See* Chapter 7 for more about the role that fruits (and vegetables) play in healthy eating and healthy weight.

What Counts as a Serving?

A one-cup serving of fruit is equal to one cup of sliced fruit, one-half cup of dried fruit, or a piece of whole fruit about the size of a tennis ball.

Fruit juice counts as part of the Fruit group (as long as it is 100 percent juice). However, since fruit juice does not contain fiber like whole and cut-up fruit, you'll want to offer less to kids. Serve preschoolers no more than one-half to three-quarters of a cup (4 to 6 ounces) of 100 percent fruit juice a day. Older kids should have no more than 8 to 12 ounces a day.

Note that fruit drinks, punch, and "ade" drinks (such as lemonade) are *not* considered part of the Fruit group because they contain mostly sugar and only a little fruit (*see* Chapter 5).

How Many Servings Do Kids Need Each Day?

The recommended number of daily fruit servings depends on a child's or teen's daily calorie needs. To find out how much fruit (in cups) your child or teen should be eating, check the Fruits column on their MyPlate daily food plan *(www.ChooseMyPlate.gov)* or see Appendixes A and B of this book.

Go For It *Fruits: Focus on Fruits*

All fresh, canned, frozen, and dried fruits are part of the Fruit group. They can be whole, cut up, or pureed like applesauce.

EXAMPLES OF *GO FOR IT* FRUITS

- Apples
- Apricots
- Bananas
- Berries (strawberries, blueberries, raspberries)
- Cherries
- Dried, unsweetened forms of fruits such as apricots, blueberries, and raisins
- Grapefruits
- Grapes
- Kiwi fruit
- Mangos
- Melons (cantaloupe, honeydew, watermelon)
- Mixed fruits (fruit cocktail)
- Nectarines
- Oranges
- Peaches
- Pears
- Papaya
- Pineapple
- Plums
- Tangerines
- 100% fruit juice (orange, apple, grape)

Take It Easy *Fruits*

Really, there are very few fruits that kids should not eat. However, some fruits do provide more calories than others. For healthy eating and a healthy weight, make sure your child or teen eats these fruits only occasionally, in limited portions, and only after eating all of his or her *Go for It* foods.

EXAMPLES OF *TAKE IT EASY* FRUITS

- Fruits packaged in syrup
- Dried forms of fruits with added sugar, such as banana chips, cranberries, or pineapple

---

Dairy

Key Nutrients in Dairy Foods

In addition to milk, the Dairy group includes foods made from milk that contain calcium, such as yogurt and cheese. However, certain other foods made with milk (such as butter, cream cheese, and cream) are not counted as part of the Dairy group because they lose their calcium during processing. These foods are categorized as *solid fats,* which are discussed later in this chapter.

In addition to calcium, other important nutrients provided by foods in the Dairy group are potassium, protein, and vitamin D. All milk and some yogurts are fortified with vitamin D (*see* Enriched versus Fortified: What's the Difference? on page 29). It's important for kids to eat and drink foods from this group, but way too many kids are missing the mark and coming up short. The nutrients in the Dairy group play a starring role in building strong bones and teeth in kids and adults. They also help prevent osteoporosis, a bone-thinning disease that affects millions of older adults. Milk and calcium-rich foods may not cause kids to lose weight, but consuming lower-fat and fat-free versions will help trim calories and saturated fat, which could lead to a healthier weight and a healthier heart (*see* What's the Big Fat Deal?).

Note: Some kids have trouble digesting milk (lactose intolerance). However, many of these kids can still enjoy milk and dairy foods. If you suspect your child or teen is lactose intolerant, check with your pediatrician to be sure (*see* Chapter 5).

WHAT'S THE BIG FAT DEAL?

Any type of fat has about 45 calories per teaspoon. But when it comes to health, certain fats are better than others, particularly when it comes to heart health. It's never too soon to start teaching your kids to eat heart smart. Here's the skinny on fat:

(continued)

WHAT'S THE BIG FAT DEAL? *(continued)*

The Good . . .

- *Polyunsaturated fatty acids* lower the production of total blood cholesterol as well as HDL (good) and LDL (bad) cholesterols. Main food sources are corn, safflower, soybean, sesame, and sunflower oils.
- *Monounsaturated fatty acids* lower the production of total blood cholesterol and LDL (bad) cholesterol. However, they raise the production of HDL (good) cholesterol. Main food sources are canola, nut, and olive oils.
- *Omega-3 fatty acids (EPA and DHA)* may help reduce blood clotting and prevent hardening of the arteries. Main food sources are various types of seafood—especially fatty fish, such as albacore tuna, mackerel, and salmon. Walnuts as well as soy, canola, and flaxseed oil provide alpha-linoleic acid, which the body converts to omega-3s.

The Bad and the Ugly . . .

- *Saturated fatty acids* raise blood cholesterol more than all other types of fat. Main food sources are animal-based foods, such as meat, poultry, butter, whole milk, and whole milk products. Plant-based sources are coconut, palm, and palm kernel oils.
- *Trans fatty acids* are formed when liquid fat is made hard (hydrogenated). *Trans* fats act like saturated fats and raise blood cholesterol levels. Although some *trans* fats are found naturally in food, most come from partially hydrogenated fats, which are commonly found in stick margarine, baked goods, and snack crackers and chips.

What Counts as a Serving?

A one-cup serving from the dairy group is equal to one cup of milk or yogurt, 1½ ounces of natural cheese, or 2 ounces of processed cheese.

How Many Servings Do Kids Need Each Day?

The recommended number of dairy servings per day depends on the child's or teen's daily calorie needs. To find out how many servings (in cups) your child or teen should eat, check the Dairy column on his or her MyPlate daily food plan *(www.ChooseMyPlate.gov)* or see Appendixes A and B of this book.

Go For It *Dairy Foods: Get Your Calcium-Rich Foods*

Several types of milk and many milk-based foods are *Go for It* foods. For healthy eating and a healthy weight, it's important that kids make several fat-free and low-fat milk group selections on a regular, daily basis (*see* Kid-Friendly Dairy Group Tips on page 40).

EXAMPLES OF *GO FOR IT* DAIRY FOODS

- Fat-free (skim) or low-fat (1%) milk
- Lactose-free milk made with fat-free or low-fat milk
- Any hard or soft cheese made with fat-free or low-fat milk
- Plain fat-free or low-fat yogurt

KID-FRIENDLY DAIRY GROUP TIPS

Here are a few pointers to help your kid enjoy the great taste of fat-free and low-fat dairy foods:

- *Start young.* After children turn two years old, you can stop offering them whole milk (they don't need the extra calories any more) and introduce them to low-fat and fat-free milk. They provide the same amount of calcium and vitamin D but with less fat, less saturated fat, and fewer calories than whole milk.
- *Break the fat habit.* To get older kids to drink fat-free milk, make the switch gradually. If they drink whole milk, try reduced fat milk, then low-fat milk, and finally fat-free milk.
- *Follow the "milk only" rule.* Make it a policy to serve fat-free or low-fat milk as the only beverages at meals.
- *Trade places.* Make macaroni and cheese, pizza, tacos, and toasted cheese sandwiches with a tasty, lower fat version of a type of cheese that your child or teen already enjoys.
- *Get cheesy with it.* Sprinkle shredded fat-free or low-fat cheese over tossed green salads, steamed broccoli, chili, and baked potatoes.
- *Make yogurt go undercover.* Substitute plain fat-free or low-fat yogurt for sour cream in any recipe or dish, such as on a baked potato.
- *Whip up a yogurt smoothie.* Blend plain fat-free or low-fat yogurt and milk with fresh berries and ice for a refreshing, nutrient-rich smoothie.
- *Keep yogurt calories to a minimum.* Many types of yogurt have added sugar between 70 and 190 calories—even if the yogurt is low fat or fat free. Compare Nutrition Facts labels to choose yogurts with less than 100 calories per serving, and choose types that are either plain or sweetened with low-calorie sweeteners.

Take It Easy *Dairy Foods*

Many of the foods and beverages in the Dairy group have added sugar and solid fat (you may not see it, but it's there!). For healthy eating and a healthy weight, make sure your child or teen eats and or drinks *Take It Easy* dairy foods only occasionally, in very limited portions, and only after eating all of his or her *Go for It* foods.

EXAMPLES OF *TAKE IT EASY* DAIRY FOODS

- Reduced-fat (2%) or whole milk
- Lactose-free milk made with reduced-fat or whole milk
- Flavored milks (such as chocolate or strawberry)
- Hard natural cheeses such as cheddar, Swiss, and Parmesan
- Soft cheeses like ricotta and cottage cheese made with reduced-fat or whole milk
- American cheese, cheese spreads, and other processed cheese
- All sugar-sweetened yogurts
- All yogurts make with reduced-fat or whole milk
- Frozen yogurt
- Ice cream
- Puddings made with sugar

Protein Foods

Key Nutrients in Protein Foods

Many foods are part of the Protein Foods group. In addition to meat and beans, this group includes poultry, fish, eggs, nuts, and seeds. As the name of the group indicates, these foods all have protein in common. Growing kids need protein to help them build and repair cells, enzymes, and hormones, and, as a last resort, to provide energy. In addition to protein, foods in the Protein Foods group supply varying amounts of zinc, magnesium, B vitamins (thiamin, niacin, vitamins B-6 and B-12), and vitamin E. Many also provide iron. The type in meat, poultry, and fish *(heme iron)* is better absorbed than the iron in eggs, dried beans, and peas *(nonheme iron)*. And while we are on the topic of health, this food group offers the max in terms of a vitamin-mineral package. For example, B vitamins act like sparkplugs to help the body use and produce energy. Protein foods also help form new blood cells and body tissues, and they help the nervous system function properly. Their iron helps carry oxygen in the blood and prevents anemia; their magnesium aids in bone building and energy release in muscles; and their zinc helps the immune system function. With that kind of nutritional boost from the foods in this group, most kids really don't need to take multivitamin supplements as long as they eating a balance of foods from all food groups (*see* Do Kids Need Multivitamins?).

DO KIDS NEED MULTIVITAMINS?

Most healthy kids do not need a multivitamin supplement. Instead, a wise selection of nutrient-rich foods is generally the best strategy for helping kids meet their nutritional needs. That's because the research suggests that foods and food patterns, and not individual nutrients, are most effective in promoting health and preventing disease. One exception may be vitamin D. Older children who drink less than four cups per day of milk fortified with vitamin D and teens who get less than 400 IU of vitamin D per day from food sources may need a vitamin D supplement. Before kids pop any supplement pills into their mouth, always check with your pediatrician or registered dietitian.

What Counts as a Serving?

A one-ounce equivalent from the Protein Foods Group is equal to one ounce of meat, poultry, or seafood; one egg; one tablespoon of peanut butter; one-half ounce of nuts or seeds; or one-fourth cup of beans or peas. (You may recall learning about beans in the Vegetable group. Nutritionally speaking, they're a double agent! They can fit in both the Protein Foods and Vegetable groups. Just be sure to count them *once* in your child's or teen's

MyPlate daily food plan—either as a serving from the Vegetable group or a serving from the Protein Foods group.)

How Many Servings Do Kids Need Each Day?

The recommended number of servings (in ounce-equivalents) that your kid should eat will depend on his or her daily calorie needs. To find out how many servings your child or teen should eat, check the Protein Foods column on his or her MyPlate daily food plan *(www.ChooseMyPlate.gov)* or see Appendixes A and B of this book.

Go for It *Protein Foods: Go Lean with Protein*

Go for It protein foods focus on choices that are low in fat (beans, peas, the leanest cuts of meat and poultry) as well as those that provide healthy oils (fish, nuts, and seeds). Choose protein foods that contain healthy oils more frequently than meat and poultry.

EXAMPLES OF *GO FOR IT* PROTEIN FOODS

- Beans and peas: all the varieties listed in *Go for It* Vegetables; processed soy products like tofu (bean curd made from soybeans), tempeh, and soy burgers/crumbles
- Beef: *lean* cuts including round steaks and roasts, top loin, sirloin, chuck shoulder, and arm roasts
- Eggs
- Ground meat or ground poultry that is 90% lean or greater
- Nuts and seeds such as almonds, cashews, peanuts, peanut butter (without added sugar or fat), pecans, pumpkin seeds, sunflower seeds, walnuts
- Pork: *lean* cuts, including pork loin, tenderloin, center loin, ham and Canadian bacon
- Poultry: skinless chicken, skinless turkey
- Seafood: most fish and shellfish
- Veal: most types

Take It Easy *Protein Foods*

Protein foods on the *Take It Easy* list provide lots of calories and contain a great deal of solid fat. For healthy eating and a healthy weight, make sure your child or teen eats them only occasionally, in very limited portions, and only after eating all of his or her *Go for It* foods.

EXAMPLES OF *TAKE IT EASY* PROTEIN FOODS

- Bacon
- Beef sausage
- Bologna
- Chicken with skin
- Ground meat or poultry that is less than 90% lean
- Hot dogs
- Peanut butter with added fat and sugar
- Pork sausage
- Salami
- Spare ribs (beef, pork, or veal)
- Turkey with skin

Oils

Key Nutrients in Oils

Oils are fats that are liquid at room temperature. They come primarily from plant sources (vegetables, nuts, and seeds) and fish.

While oils are not considered a MyPlate food group, kids do need a small amount each day for good health. Oils are the body's main source of vitamin E (a powerful antioxidant) as well as a major source of monounsaturated fatty acids (MUFA) and polyunsaturated fatty acids (PUFA), which are both considered good fats because they don't raise blood cholesterol (*see* What's the Big Fat Deal? on page 37). PUFA also contain essential fatty acids that are necessary for a healthy nervous system and skin.

What Counts as a Serving?

Daily recommendations for oils are measured in teaspoons. One teaspoon of oil is equal to one teaspoon of vegetable oil (canola, olive, corn, etc.).

One ounce of nuts or seeds provides about three teaspoons of oil. Salad dressings, mayonnaise, and soft margarines provide about 2½ teaspoons of oil per tablespoon.

How Much Oil Do Kids Need Each Day?

Most kids consume enough oil in the foods they eat, such as fish, nuts, and salad dressing. The recommended daily limits are based on a kid's daily calorie needs. Check the Know Your Limits section of your child's or teen's MyPlate daily food plan *(www.ChooseMyPlate.gov)* for the recommended daily limit on oils (in teaspoons) or see Appendixes A and B of this book.

Go for It *Oils*

The list of *Go for It* oils includes healthy oils as well as certain foods that also provide oils. Keep in mind that healthy oils still provide a lot of calories (45 calories per teaspoon or 135 calories per tablespoon). The best way to help your child or teen achieve a healthy weight is to replace solid fats with oils, instead of eating oils in addition to fats!

EXAMPLES OF *GO FOR IT* OILS

- Fish: tuna, salmon
- Healthy oils: canola, corn, cottonseed, olive, safflower, sesame, soybean, sunflower, walnut
- Mayonnaise
- Nuts and seeds: all types
- Olives
- Soft (tub or squeeze) margarine with no *trans* fats

Take It Easy *Oils*

Although the *Take It Easy* oils come from plants, they provide more saturated fat (which raises blood cholesterol) than MUFA or PUFA. Check food labels as these oils are in many foods, like crackers, cookies, and even popcorn (*see* Chapter 9).

EXAMPLES OF *TAKE IT EASY* OILS

- Coconut oil
- Palm oil
- Palm kernel oil

Solid Fats and Added Sugar— Cut Way Back or Cut It Out!

You may have noticed that certain foods and beverages are missing from the five food groups and oils. That's because they are high in solid fat, added sugar, and calories while not providing nutrients that kids need. To eat healthy and be a healthy weight, kids should take it easy on these "extras" and stay within the calorie limits listed in the Know Your Limits section of their MyPlate daily food plan.

EXAMPLES OF *TAKE IT EASY* SOLID FAT AND ADDED SUGAR FOODS

- Sugar-sweetened beverages: regular soda, fruit drinks, fruit punch
- Solid fats: butter, shortening, stick margarine
- Hydrogenated oils
- Candy
- Cream cheese
- Dessert topping
- Gravy
- Heavy whipping cream

Combination Foods

Where do foods that combine multiple food groups, like pizza, tacos, and lasagna, fit in your kid's daily food plan? An easy way to find out is to use MyFood-a-pedia, which is available on the MyPlate Web site *(www .choosemyplate.gov)* and as a Web tool optimized for cellphones *(www .MyFoodapedia.gov)*. When you enter the food and the serving size that was eaten, the tool automatically shows all the food groups in the food and the amounts of each to count in the daily food plan. For example, for one beef taco with cheese, lettuce, and tomato, MyFood-a-pedia calculates the food groups and amounts to be:

- Grains group: 1 ounce
- Vegetable group: ¼ cup
- Protein Foods group: 1 ounce
- Dairy group: ¼ cup

How to Plan Healthy and Balanced Meals

Now that you know what *types* of healthy food your family needs to eat as well as the *amounts*, let's put the pieces together and come up with a *Healthy Eating, Healthy Weight* daily meal plan. Remember that each family member will need a personalized plan to match his or her specific nutrient needs. If your child is older than two years, the MyPlate Web site *(www.choosemyplate.gov)* can help you determine a daily food plan that's right for your son or daughter.

> **Parents Weigh In: MyPlate Food Planner Fan**
>
> I *love* the MyPlate planner! It helps me keep on track with my goal to plan healthy menus for my family. It also saves me so much time. I use it every Sunday night to plan menus for the week.
>
> —ANNE, MOTHER OF TWO KIDS UNDER THE AGE OF FOUR

Calories Count

Before you can select a MyPlate daily food plan, you need to know how many calories your child or teen needs each day. You can find this information on the MyPlate Web site, or refer to Appendix A of this book. Also, if you need help "guess-timating" your child's physical activity level, here are a few guidelines (*see* Chapter 4 for more help):

- *Sedentary* = less than 30 minutes of moderate physical activity a day.
- *Moderately active* = between 30 and 60 minutes of moderate physical activity a day.
- *Active* = 60 or more minutes of moderate physical activity a day.

Remember the Jackson family described at the start of the chapter? Assuming the kids are sedentary, here's how many calories each would need:

- 13-year-old Anthony: 2,000 calories per day
- 8-year-old Kendra: 1,400 calories per day
- 4-year-old Keeshawn: 1,200 calories per day

How many calories does your son or daughter need? Check out the MyPlate Web site or Appendix A and write your answer here: _____ calories per day.

How to Pick a MyPlate Daily Food Plan

Once you know your child's or teen's daily calorie level, you can quickly determine his or her MyPlate daily food plan. MyPlate offers 12 daily food plans with recommended amounts of food to eat from the five basic food groups and oils category to meet your child's or teen's healthy eating and healthy weight requirements. (For copies of these plans, *see* Appendix B at the back of this book).

Again, using the Jackson family as our example, we've created a chart showing the MyPlate daily food plans for each child.

What does your kid's MyPlate daily food plan look like? To determine your child's or teen's MyPlate daily food plan, turn to Appendix B in this book. Alternatively, go to the MyPlate Web site *(www.ChooseMyPlate*

MYPLATE DAILY FOOD PLANS FOR THE JACKSON FAMILY

	Keeshawn	Kendra	Anthony
Calorie level	1,200	1,400	2,000
Grains	4 ounce-equivalents	5 ounce-equivalents	6 ounce-equivalents
Vegetables	1½ cups	1½ cups	2½ cups
Fruits	1 cup	1½ cups	2 cups
Dairy	2 cups	2 cups	3 cups
Protein foods	3 ounce-equivalents	4 ounce-equivalents	5½ ounce-equivalents
Oil	4 teaspoons	4 teaspoons	6 teaspoons
Maximum amount of calories from solid fats and added sugars	171	171	267

.gov) and enter your child's gender, age, and activity level. The site will automatically generate a customized MyPlate daily food plan that you can print. While you're on the site, you can print a plan for yourself, too!

MyPlate Daily Meal Plan in Action

Now that you know which food groups your family needs to eat and the recommended portions, you have the tools to start building *Healthy Eating, Healthy Weight* menus that your whole family can enjoy. To get you started, we're providing an example for the Jackson kids. Notice that Keeshawn's servings are often smaller than those of his older sister and brother. You can find many other menu ideas in Chapter 11.

SAMPLE ONE-DAY HEALTHY EATING, HEALTHY WEIGHT MENU FOR THE JACKSON FAMILY

	Serving Sizes		
Menu	Keeshawn	Kendra	Anthony
Breakfast: Oatmeal with bananas			
• Whole grain oats	1 cup	1 cup	1 cup
• Banana slices	¼ cup	½ cup	½ cup
• Low-fat milk	½ cup	½ cup	½ cup
Lunch: Chicken sandwich topped with veggies			
• Whole wheat bread	1 slice	1 slice	2 slices
• Low-fat American cheese	½ ounce	½ ounce	1 ounce
• Sliced chicken	1 ounce	1 ounce	2 ounces
• Grated carrots	¼ cup	¼ cup	¼ cup
• Baby spinach	½ cup	½ cup	½ cup
• Diced cantaloupe	¼ cup	½ cup	½ cup
Dinner: Rice and beans with sausage			
• Brown rice	½ cup	1 cup	1 cup
• Black beans	¼ cup	¼ cup	¼ cup
• Turkey sausage	1 ounce	2 ounces	2½ ounces
• Bell pepper	¼ cup	¼ cup	¼ cup
• Broccoli	¼ cup	¼ cup	¼ cup
• Low-fat milk	½ cup	½ cup	1 cup
Snack 1: Stuffed Pita Pocket			
• Baked whole wheat pita	½ pita	½ pita	1 pita
• Tomato salsa	¼ cup	¼ cup	½ cup
• Sugar snap peas	¼ cup	¼ cup	½ cup
Snack 2: Fruit smoothie			
• Berries	½ cup	½ cup	1 cup
• Low-fat milk	¼ cup	¼ cup	½ cup
• Low-fat yogurt	¼ cup	¼ cup	½ cup

Snacks—An Important Part of Healthy Eating

Preschoolers have tiny tummy capacities. Teens are eating machines. Three daily meals may not be enough to provide all the nutrients kids require. Because many kids need to eat snacks to help them grow properly and to fill any nutritional gaps, snacks are an important part of your child's or teen's MyPlate daily food plan.

On the other hand, snacking has received a bad rap—and rightly so! Today's on-the-go family lifestyle interferes with sit-down family meals (*see* Chapter 10), and as a consequence some kids snack up to six times a day. This sort of frequent snacking is called "grazing," and it may cause some kids to overeat. In fact, kids between the ages of 2 and 18 are getting about 526 calories a day from snacks, which is roughly a 200-calorie-a-day increase compared to a decade ago. Multiply 200 calories by 365 days, and you're looking at a weight gain of 20 pounds in a year. Yikes! To make snacking matters even worse, kids are no longer munching on apples and sipping milk. Nowadays, they generally snack on foods like cookies and soft drinks that provide extra calories from added sugar and solid fat.

So, does snacking really cause kids to be overweight? At this time, most research indicates unhealthy weight gain is not related to *how often* kids snack, but it does seem to be related to *what* they are snacking on and *how much* they eat or drink. For this reason, we encourage you to note the difference between a snack and a treat. *Snacks* are everyday foods and should come from MyPlate *Go for It* choices. *Treats* are once-in-a-while foods and often come from MyPlate *Take It Easy* choices. The key to smart snacking is planning: offer your kids healthy snacks at regularly scheduled times. To help you teach your kids healthy snacking habits, here are some guidelines that address the five essential "W's": *who* should snack, *why* kids should

---

Kids Weigh In: MyPlate Food Tracker Fan

When my registered dietitian showed me how to use the MyPlate food tracker, I was so surprised to learn how many calories I was getting from just my snacks. I have been using the tracker for a few weeks, and it really helps me keep track of my calories each day!

—NICOLE, AGE 15

snack, *when* kids should snack, *where* kids should snack, and *what* they should snack on for a healthy weight. Make sure that you share these snack guidelines with everyone who cares for your child or teen—babysitters, daycare, school, and especially relatives.

Who *Should Snack?*

No restrictions here. Most kids of all ages need to snack. Even if kids are overweight, a healthy snack can fit into their daily eating plan.

Why *Should Kids Snack?*

At each age and stage of growing up, kids need snacks. Here are some of the reasons.

Preschoolers

Preschoolers are, of course, much smaller than adults, but pound-for-pound their total calorie needs are comparable. Young children's stomachs are not large enough to get enough calories from only three meals a day. They're like cars with small gas tanks. They need refueling throughout the day.

Children Ages 5 to 12

Kids in this age group need snacks to help them grow and learn. Early school lunch hours followed by a long stretch before dinner can leave children and tweens running on empty. Kids who eat balanced snacks pay better attention in class, make fewer mistakes on tests, and generally have fewer behavior problems.

Teenagers

During the teen years, calorie needs are at an all-time high, especially for boys. Rapid growth spurts, intense sports workouts, and staying up later at night leave teens ravenous. It's no wonder they have snack attacks.

When *Should Kids Snack?*

Unplanned, random snacking can lead to problems, especially with weight. Nonstop snacking interferes with kids' appetites and can disrupt their natural instinct to experience hunger and fullness (*see* Hungry or Satisfied? on page 54). On the other hand, snacks can actually help kids achieve a healthy weight when they are timed correctly. Most children and teens need to eat every three to four hours throughout the day to meet their MyPlate daily food plan. This translates into the following:

- Younger kids need to eat three meals and at least two snacks a day.
- Older kids need to eat three meals and at least one snack a day (they may need two snacks if they're going through a growth spurt or if they are very physically active).

Parents and caregivers need to offer planned meals and snacks consistently throughout the day. A good rule of thumb is to offer snacks a few hours after one meal ends and about one to two hours before the next meal begins. Postponing snacks until a few hours after a meal helps prevent kids from refusing food at a meal and then begging for more food as a "snack" just after the meal ends. On the other hand, putting a stop to snacking immediately before meals encourages a healthy appetite at mealtimes. Above all, remember the bottom line: if snacks are planned, coordinated with meals, and served consistently at regularly scheduled times, kids are more likely to be a healthy weight.

Where *Should Kids Snack?*

When at home, designate a certain area as the "eating-only zone" and limit all snacking to that location. The kitchen table or countertop works well. When kids snack all over the house, that makes it hard for you to monitor what and how much they're eating. (Plus, all the crumbs and spills can get messy!) Also, never let kids eat snacks while watching television. Studies show that this mindless munching leads to overeating, which often results in unhealthy weight gain (*see* Chapter 4)

HUNGRY OR SATISFIED?

To become healthy eaters, kids need to listen to their bodies. You can help your child or teen tune in to his or her tummy (appetite awareness) by using the 10-point hunger scale described below. Before and after eating, ask your son or daughter to choose the number that matches how he or she feels. Then teach them how to get into the "zones" between 3 and 6.

Hunger Scale

Feeling	Zone
1 **Empty**: You feel light-headed and weak from not eating all day. 2 **Starving**: You feel cranky and can't concentrate.	**Danger Zone**: Be careful not to overeat. Better yet—stay out of this zone!
3 **Hungry**: Your tummy is rumbling with hunger pangs. 4 **Slightly hungry**: You're just starting to feel hungry.	**Eating Zone**: You're physically hungry. Time to eat!
5 **Neutral**: You're not hungry or full. 6 **Perfectly comfortable**: You feel satisfied.	**Stop Eating Zone**: You're satisfied. Put down the fork and walk away from the table.
7 **Full**: You feel slightly uncomfortable. 8 **Uncomfortably full**: You feel bloated. 9 **Stuffed**: Your cloths are too tight and you can't move. 10 **Overstuffed**: You are about to puke.	**Red Alert Zone**: Since you are totally full, chances are you're *emotionally* hungry—bored, lonely, anxious, sad, happy, tired, etc.

What *Should Kids Eat for Snacks?*

When selecting snacks, use your son's or daughter's MyPlate daily food plan as your guide. First, consider what your child or teen typically eats at meals. The My Daily Food Plan Worksheet, which you can download from the MyPlate Web site *(www.ChooseMyPlate.gov),* can help you quickly evaluate how what your kid actually eats compares to his or her customized MyPlate daily food plan. If your kid is falling short in certain food groups, snack time is a great time to fill in the gaps with *Go for It* foods. For example, if your child needs more vegetables or dairy foods, offer baby carrots and yogurt dip for a snack.

Another thing you'll want to consider is the nutrient composition of the snack. Snacks that contain a mixture of carbohydrate, protein, and fat (such as peanut butter and celery, or fruit and yogurt) will satisfy hunger for a longer time than a snack with only carbohydrate (such as fruit or pretzels). The mixed-nutrient snacks are therefore a better choice when there's going to be a long interval between meals. On the other hand, if you need to offer a snack shortly before a meal to take the edge off hunger, it's better to provide a snack that is mostly carbohydrate (*Go for It* fruits, grains, and vegetables).

And, of course, the size of the snack also matters. A good starting point for snack portions is the recommended serving sizes in MyPlate (*see* Chapter 6). Also remember to choose servings that fit within your kid's daily plan for all meals and snacks.

Quick, Easy, and Balanced Snacks

As you plan snacks, be creative and get the kids involved. Here are some kid-friendly snack ideas that include at least two food groups. You can also find snack recipes in Chapter 11 and on our Web site *(www.HealthyEatingForFamilies.com).*

- Whole grain cereal and fat-free milk
- Fruit smoothie (100 percent fruit juice blended with low-fat or fat-free milk or yogurt)
- Fat-free plain yogurt and fresh berries
- Low-fat peanut butter (no added sugar) on whole wheat crackers

- Whole wheat pita and hummus (chickpea dip)
- Apple or pear slices topped with low-fat cheese
- Oven-baked bagel chips and salsa
- Dried cranberry and peanut mix
- Whole wheat pita stuffed with lettuce, tomato, cucumber, and low-fat dressing
- Raw veggies dipped in fat-free ranch dressing blended with plain, low-fat yogurt
- Plain microwave popcorn and 100 percent fruit juice
- Quesadilla (whole wheat soft tortilla and low-fat cheese, folded and heated)
- Flaked tuna or salmon and chopped celery, with low-fat mayonnaise
- Microwave-baked potato topped with salsa and shredded low-fat cheese
- One cup of tomato soup (made with low-fat or fat-free milk) and whole grain crackers

Healthy Meals: Menus for Three Weeks

By this point in the chapter, we hope you feel inspired and prepared to start a *Healthy Eating, Healthy Weight* daily meal plan for your family. At the same time, you're probably also aware that your family needs some time to master eating regularly scheduled meals and snacks that are balanced and healthy. Just keep in mind that the effort will pay off! To help you get started, in Chapter 11 you'll find family-friendly recipes and three weeks' worth of daily menus (because, as we noted in Chapter 2, it takes about three weeks to establish a new behavior pattern). When adapting the menus for your family, use each person's MyPlate daily food plan to determine the serving sizes. Bon appétit!

Healthy Eating, Healthy Weight—You're in Control

■ *Keeshawn's clinic visit was a wake-up call for the entire Jackson family. Even Gramma agreed that they all needed to eat healthier. As a family, they sat down and wrote a contract that identified the* Healthy Eating, Healthy Weight *goals they would work on:*

> *We, the Jackson family, will work toward the following goals over the next one or two weeks: (1) Use the MyPlate Food Planner to plan family meals for the week (and stick with the menu). (2) Follow a meal and snack schedule. (3) Sit at the kitchen table or counter for all meals and snacks (with the TV off). When we have successfully made these a habit, we will reward ourselves with a trip to the beach.* Signed *Elizabeth Jackson, Anthony Jackson, Kendra Jackson, and Keeshawn Jackson.*

True to the contract, Elizabeth printed MyPlate daily food plans for the kids and herself. She searched for quick and healthy recipes online and used the MyPlate Food Planner to plan her family meals. On Saturdays, she and Keeshawn now go to the grocery store or local farmer's market. Keeshawn loves looking at the fresh produce and tasting samples. Last visit he tried kiwi and fresh pineapple. Elizabeth and Gramma set up a meal and snack schedule for Keeshawn and enforced the rule that he has to sit at the kitchen counter to eat and the TV must be turned off. The older kids have enjoyed learning about MyPlate. Kendra uses the My Daily Food Planner Worksheet to keep track of her own daily eating. Elizabeth hangs it on the refrigerator next to Keeshawn's worksheet. Anthony likes the MyPlate Food Tracker; he uses the computer at his afterschool program to check his progress. When Elizabeth is too busy at work to prepare a home-cooked meal, she now stops by the grocery store for a deli-roasted chicken "deal meal" with the vegetable fixings. All in all, everyone feels healthier. ■

Today's on-the-go lifestyle has many families eating meals on the fly, and this may be one of the key reasons that kids' weights are skyrocketing. But kids are more likely to be a healthy weight when their families consistently apply *Healthy Eating, Healthy Weight Strategy #1: Eat with a plan! Enjoy delicious family meals and snacks that are balanced and healthy.*

It is time for your family to come up with some goals related to this *Healthy Eating, Healthy Weight* strategy. After your family has decided together on a few goals, write them down as a goal contract like the one found at the end of Chapter 2. Remember to have everyone show their commitment by signing the contract. Here are some examples of possible goals to get your family started:

- Use the MyPlate Food Planner to plan family meals for the week (and stick with the menu).
- Follow a meal and snack schedule.
- Limit snacks to set times of the day.
- Sit down on Sunday and make a healthy snack menu for the week.
- Eat meals and snacks only at the kitchen table.
- Switch to low-fat milk, yogurt, and cheese
- Make half of our daily grain choices whole grain.
- Use the MyPlate Food Tracker daily to help me eat healthier.

At the end of the week, sit down and track your family's progress. Use a tracking sheet like the one at the end of Chapter 2 to score your family's progress toward your goals. Once you feel you have mastered the goal(s), move on to another goal. You may also be ready to tackle another *Healthy Eating, Healthy Weight* strategy. Don't forget to reward your family and celebrate your successes.

4

Healthy Eating, Healthy Weight Strategy #2: Turn Off the Tube and Move!

■ *Twelve-year-old Samantha Davis loves being a tween. Now that she is in middle school, she has many friends. Although she doesn't see them much, they stay connected by computer and cellphone. In fact, Samantha spends several hours a day sitting in front of a screen—downloading and listening to music, texting, chatting online, watching television, and playing video games. While she's "plugged in," she sips sodas and grazes on chips and candy. All this media-multitasking leaves little time for Samantha to rollerblade and be as active as she used to be. Her grades have gone down, too. On her last report card, she even received a "D" in physical education. When asked about this grade, Samantha said, "I hate gym. It's embarrassing changing in front of other kids, and I don't want to get all sweaty." Her parents have noticed that Samantha has gained a lot of weight in the past year so they talked with her PE teacher to find out how they could encourage Samantha to be more active. The teacher recommended that they help Samantha by becoming more physically active as a family. More specifically, he recom-mended Healthy Eating, Healthy Weight Strategy #2: Turn off the tube and move! Limit all screen time to less than two hours a day and be physically active 60 minutes or more a day.* ■

Jack LaLanne, Jane Fonda, Richard Simmons, Jillian Michaels—every era has its workout icons. But do you know who is the most influential exercise role model for your child or teen? It's you! Kids are more likely to limit TV and other screen time if you do, and if they have fun family activities to enjoy. So, to encourage your child or teen to be more physically active, give *Healthy Eating, Healthy Weight Strategy #2* a try. Studies have found that kids who regularly participate in physical activity are less likely to be overweight. In addition, reducing inactivity (screen time) seems to help in treating and preventing unhealthy weight gain. If Samantha, our high-tech tween, reminds you of your son or daughter, keep reading. This chapter will help you "unplug" your kid and motivate him or her to engage in fun physical activity for at least 60 minutes every day.

Inter-Inactive Kids

Inactivity among American children and teens is alarmingly high. According to the Centers for Disease Control and Prevention, during nonschool hours, almost two-thirds of kids between the ages of 9 and 13 years do not participate in any organized physical activity and about one-quarter do not engage in any free-time physical activity. As kids get older, they tend to become even less physically active. In 2009 only 18 percent of high school students participated in at least 60 minutes of physical activity each day, and only 23 percent attended physical education class daily. And, according to the 2010 Dietary Guidelines for Americans, less than half of kids between the ages of 12 and 21 years exercise on a daily basis.

Why should these statistics worry us? Because the evidence is clear: regular physical activity promotes health and fitness in children and teens. Compared to kids who are inactive, physically active kids tend to be more physically fit, have stronger bones and muscles, and feel better about themselves—they may even have reduced symptoms of anxiety and depression. They also have a lower risk of developing heart disease, colon cancer, and type 2 diabetes. Furthermore, regular physical activity helps kids of all ages with weight control. In fact, when it comes to a healthy weight being physically active is just as important for kids as eating right. Regular physical activity helps control the percentage of body fat in children and teens. Studies have shown that overweight and obese kids can reduce their body fat by participating in 30 to 60 minutes of moderately intense physical activity, three to five days a week.

Media Alert! Excessive Screen Time May Be Hazardous to Kids' Weight

So why aren't more American kids outside running, riding bikes, and shooting hoops? The answer may be too much electronic competition. Kids spend hours sitting in school, and then they come home and sit for additional hours as they do homework, chat online with friends, text, play video games, or watch TV. Thanks to an explosion in mobile and online media, kids can stay wired 24/7, and statistics show that kids between the ages of 8 and 18 devote about 7½ hours a day to using electronic media. Oftentimes, they are simultaneously using multiple types of media equipment, such as a cellphone, an MP3 player, and a laptop, so they actually manage to squeeze in almost 11 hours worth of media content into those 7½ hours! And older kids aren't the only ones zoning out in front of a TV screen. Preschoolers are also spending more time watching than playing and being active. A KidsHealth survey *(www.kidshealth.org)* found that children under the age of 6 watch an average of about two hours of screen media a day, primarily TV and videos or DVDs.

In addition to being inactive, kids often snack when they're in front of a screen (a TV or computer), in part because they are enticed by a steady diet of junk food ads. Put these ingredients together, and you have a recipe for weight gain.

Healthy Eating, Healthy Weight Strategy #2 therefore involves limiting kids' screen time to a maximum of two hours a day. Why two hours? Although watching TV and playing video games may not cause kids to become overweight, several studies have found a strong link between screen time and weight gain. One study found that among 12- to 17-year-olds, the prevalence of obesity increased by 2 percent for each additional hour of television kids viewed. Other studies discovered that youth who watch more than five hours of TV a day are much more likely to be overweight than kids who watch one hour or less. Also, while the verdict is still out, some preliminary studies suggest that "zoning out" in front of a TV screen may lower kids' metabolism, which would mean they need fewer calories each day and are at risk of gaining extra weight.

Is Your Child Wired?

Where does your child or teen fit into the multimedia picture? How much time does your preschooler spend in front of a screen? If you're not sure, it's time to find out. Challenge everyone in the family to keep a week-long log of how much time they spend watching TV or DVDs, listening to music, on a computer and the Internet, and using a cellphone. You can download a screen-time log from the National Heart Lung and Blood Institute's We Can! program Web site (www.nhlbi.nih.gov/health/public /heart/obesity/wecan/reduce-screen-time/index .htm) or create a simple tracking sheet using pen and paper. Then take a look at the daily totals. If your child's or teen's screen time is less than two hours a day, congratulations! If it's more than two hours, keep reading.

> **Kids Weigh In: Better Report Cards**
>
> After Dad moved the computer out of my bedroom, my grades improved *and* I found that I like seeing my family more.
> —ALEX, AGE 14

Screen Time, Mindless Munching, and Food Ads

In addition to deterring kids from being physically active, watching TV and playing computer games promotes overeating. For starters, many kids like to eat in front of a screen. However, it takes about 20 minutes for the brain to signal the stomach that it is full, which means kids can easily polish off a big bag of potato chips as they watch their favorite cartoon without being aware of what they're doing. In addition, kids are bombarded with commercials that encourage them to eat high-calorie foods loaded with added sugar and fat. The average child sees about 40,000 TV ads each year, and most of the ads targeted to kids are for candy, cereal, soft drinks, snack chips, and fast food. In fact, one study found that if kids (or adults) ate a 2,000 calorie diet consisting entirely of foods advertised on TV, they would consume 25 times the recommended daily servings of sugars and 20 times the recommended servings of fat. However, the advertised foods would provide fewer than half the recommended servings of vegetables, dairy products, and fruit.

As every parent who has ever taken a child grocery shopping knows, kids want the foods they see advertised on TV. Preschoolers are particularly vulnerable to food ads. Studies have repeatedly shown that kids between the ages of four and six years think foods taste better when their favorite cartoon character is on the package or TV screen. Here are some tips to help you wean your child or teen off a steady stream of junk food commercials.

- *Make a family rule to not eat while watching TV shows or videos.* This policy should apply to watching anything on a TV, computer screen, or other electronic device. When it's time for a snack, turn off the screen and let kids munch on fresh fruit or veggies and low-fat dip at the kitchen table or their designated eating area. (For more healthy snack ideas, *see* Chapter 3.)
- *Record programs for younger kids and view them without the advertisements.* Kids under the age of eight years don't understand that commercials sell products. Up to the age of six years, children are unable to distinguish program content from commercials, especially if their favorite character is promoting the product. Even older kids may need to be reminded of the purpose of advertising.
- *Buy or rent children's DVDs.* Be sure to fast-forward through any advertisements that appear at the beginning of the video.
- *Encourage kids to watch public television stations.* Although some public TV programs are sponsored by companies, the products they sell are rarely shown.
- *Keep tabs on food ads.* Help your family tune-in to food marketing. For a few days, have your older child or teen write down the types of foods and beverages advertised on shows that the family watches. When everyone's done, review the logs together and answer the following questions: What types of foods were advertised the most? How often do you eat these foods in a week? What types of foods

were advertised the least? How often do you eat these foods in a week?

Kids Unplugged

Whether your child is in preschool or high school, one thing is for certain—it is time for you to seize the remote and take control. Reducing the amount of time your child or teen spends with media will have a positive impact on his or her weight—even if eating habits do not otherwise change. In studies, a 10-day "turn-off" period followed by a seven-hour weekly limit on screen time seems to help kids decrease their body mass index and body fat. Here are a few pointers to help you disconnect your child or teen from the screen:

- *Take the media out of the bedroom.* Today, 71 percent of all kids ages 8 to 18 years have their own TVs in their rooms. In addition, 50 percent have a video game player or cable TV, and 30 percent have a computer and Internet access in their bedrooms. Kids with a TV in their bedroom watch about 1½ hours more a day than kids who don't have one in their bedroom.
- *Eat electronic-free meals.* Make it a family rule to turn off the TV while eating and make sure that everybody docks their cellphones so you can talk with each other.
- *Try a weekday ban.* Record favorite weekday shows and save TV time for the weekends. Watch shows as a family and fast-forward through the commercials. Remember, too, that your goal is to limit screen time to less than two hours a day—even on the weekends!
- *Pass a family screen time policy.* As a family, discuss ways to cut back on recreational screen time. Ask the kids to come up with reasonable limits; as parents, you should do the same. Then write up a contract and have everybody sign it (*see* the sample contract form at the end of Chapter 2). If the family reaches the goal, reward yourselves with a physical activity you can all enjoy, like a trip to a museum or local playground.

- *Enjoy an action-packed evening.* After dinner, resist the urge to watch TV. Take the dog for a walk; go for a family bike ride; play outdoor games like red rover, tag, duck-duck-goose, or hide-and-seek; or play active indoor games like charades, Twister, and hot potato.
- *Turn off Saturday morning cartoons.* Take kids to the local park, recreation center, or health club. Play a game of basketball, let them climb on the monkey bars, or sign them up for swimming lessons.
- *Get up and dance.* Take the headphones off, turn up the music, and have a family dance contest. Can anybody do the moonwalk or the worm?
- *Hang out with friends.* Instead of communicating by computer or cellphones, encourage older kids to get together with their friends and do something fun like walk around the mall, go sledding, or play a pick-up game of soccer. For younger kids, invite a friend over and encourage active forms of play instead of watching TV or playing video games.
- *Play interactive video games.* Invest in or rent video games that require kids to get up and move their arms and legs—no sitting allowed.
- *Make screen time an active time.* When kids do watch TV, prevent them from being a slouch on the couch. Have a contest to see who can do the most push-ups or jumping jacks during a commercial break. Older kids can stretch, do yoga, or lift weights while watching TV.

Let's Get Physical!

So far, we've focused on how the first part of *Healthy Eating, Healthy Weight Strategy #2:* limiting all screen time to less than two hours a day. Now let's take a closer look at the second part of the strategy—getting kids to move and be physically active 60 minutes or more a day.

Exercise is good for you—everyone knows that. But many of us are confused about the details: How much exercise do kids need? What types

**Parents Weigh In:
Recess Time!**

At my son's school, he eats lunch at his desk and they stopped having recess. If I had to sit at my desk at work all day long without breaks, I'd be bouncing off the walls!

JOE, DAD OF A SIX-YEAR BOY

are best to improve health and reach a healthy weight? To answer these questions, the U.S. Department of Health and Human Services issued Physical Activity Guidelines for Americans *(www.health.gov /paguidelines)* in 2008. These science-based recommendations apply to everyone six years or older and are broken down into three age groups: children and adolescents, adults, and older adults (65+ years old). Here is how they apply specifically to kids.

How Much Physical Activity Should Kids Get?

According to the Physical Activity Guidelines for Americans, children and teens should be physically active for at least 60 minutes a day. Now, if your child or teen has been spending more time texting than being active, 60 minutes may sound like eternity. However, keep in mind that kids can break the 60 minutes into shorter periods spread throughout the day. Walking to and from school, playing tag at recess, raking leaves, and a quick game of basketball in the evening—they all count toward the daily goal.

What Types of Physical Activity Do Kids Need?

While meeting their daily goal of 60 minutes or more of physical activity, kids should include each of the following three types of physical activity on at least three days a week:

- *Vigorous aerobic activities:* These kinds of activities involve rhythmic movements of large muscles (arms and legs) and get kids' hearts pumping and blood flowing. Aerobic activities can be *moderate intensity* or *vigorous intensity*. How do you measure the intensity of an activity? Imagine a scale from zero to 10, where sitting is zero intensity and the highest level of effort possible is 10. *Moderate-intensity activity* is a five or six. Kids will notice that their hearts are beating faster than normal and they are breathing harder than normal. A good example is a brisk walk to school. *Vigorous-intensity* activity is at a level of seven or eight. Kids will feel their heart beating much faster than normal, and they will be breathing much harder than normal. A good example is running on the playground. Keep in mind that children often do activities in short bursts, which may not technically be aerobic (because brief activity doesn't increase the heart rate for a long period of time). However, this activity still counts toward their daily 60 minutes.

- *Muscle-strengthening activities:* These kinds of activities make muscles do more work than they usually do during typical activities of daily life. Muscle-strengthening activities can be unstructured and part of play, such as playing on playground equipment, climbing trees, and playing tug-of-war, or they can be structured activities, such as lifting weights or working with resistance bands. Be sure to check with your pediatrician about age-specific weight-lifting guidelines before your child or teen starts a program.

- *Bone-strengthening activities:* These kinds of activities produce a force on the bones that promotes bone growth and strength. This force is commonly produced by impact with the ground.

Check out the chart titled Aerobic, Muscle-Strengthening, and Bone-Strengthening Activities (page 68) for fun, age-appropriate examples of each type of exercise. You'll notice some overlap among the categories—for example, running is both an aerobic and a bone-strengthening activity. Therefore, it can count toward your kid's daily goal of 60 minutes or more of physical activity as well the weekly goals for both bone-strengthening and aerobic activity.

Physical Activity and Preschoolers

You may have noticed that the Physical Activity Guidelines for Americans are intended for individuals age six years and older. If your child is younger, how much physical activity should he or she get each day? While there are no specific recommendations, MyPlate for Preschoolers offers some excellent guidelines and tips *(www.ChooseMyPlate.gov/Preschoolers/PhysicalActivity)*.

AEROBIC, MUSCLE-STRENGTHENING, AND BONE-STRENGTHENING ACTIVITIES

Type of Activity	Appropriate for . . .
Moderate-intensity aerobic activities	
Active recreation, such as hiking, skateboarding, or rollerblading	Children, teens
Bicycle riding	Children, teens
Brisk walking	Children, teens
Canoeing	Teens
Housework and yard work, such as sweeping or pushing a lawn mower	Teens
Games that require catching and throwing, such as baseball and softball	Teens
Vigorous-intensity aerobic activities	
Active games involving running and chasing, such as tag	Children
Active games involving running and chasing, such as flag football	Teens
Bicycle riding	Children, teens
Jumping rope	Children, teens
Martial arts, such as karate	Children, teens
Running	Children, teens
Sports such as soccer, ice or field hockey, basketball, swimming, and tennis	Children, teens
Cross-country skiing	Children, teens
Vigorous dancing	Teens
Muscle-strengthening activities	
Games such as tug-of-war	Children, teens
Modified push-ups (with knees on the floor)	Children
Push-ups and pull-ups	Teens

AEROBIC, MUSCLE-STRENGTHENING, AND BONE-STRENGTHENING ACTIVITIES *(continued)*

Type of Activity	Appropriate for . . .
Muscle-strengthening activities	
Resistance exercises using body weight or resistance bands	Children
Resistance exercises with exercise bands, weight machines, or hand-held weights	Teens
Rope or tree climbing	Children
Climbing wall	Teens
Sit-ups (curl-ups or crunches)	Children, teens
Swinging on playground equipment/bars	Children
Bone-strenghtening activities	
Games such as hopscotch	Children
Hopping, skipping, and jumping	Children, teens
Jumping rope	Children, teens
Running	Children, teens
Sports such as gymnastics, basketball, volleyball, and tennis	Children, teens

Adapted from Centers for Disease Control and Prevention. Physical Activity for Everyone. How Much Exercise Do Children Need? *www.cdc.gov/physicalactivity/everyone/guidelines/children.html.*

Generally speaking, you should encourage your preschooler to play actively several times every day. It's perfectly normal that their activity happens in short bursts of time rather than all at once. Also, keep in mind physical activity does not always have to be led by adults. Young children need plenty of "free play" time in which they engage in unstructured physical activity, use their imaginations, and get to be kids. Some examples of free play are playing on the playground, playing tag with friends, or simply chasing other kids while pretending to be wild animals. Of course, adult-led activities that are structured to have a purpose, such as encouraging flexibility, focusing on strength, or concentrating on endurance, are important, too.

How can you tell if your preschooler is getting enough physical activity? Ask yourself the following questions. If you can usually answer "yes" to these questions, your preschooler is probably getting enough physical activity.

- Does your preschooler play outdoors or in a room where they are free to run around several times a day?
- Does your preschooler watch less than two hours of TV daily (including all screen time)?
- Do you make sure that your preschooler doesn't sit for more than 60 minutes at one time?
- When actively playing, is your preschooler breathing quickly and/ or sweating?

As children grow, their motor skills and coordination improve, which expands the range of physical activities they can enjoy. Here are some general guidelines to help you determine when your preschooler may be ready for certain activities. Also, read through the Fun Physical Activities for Preschoolers for a variety of indoor and outdoor activities you can do with your preschooler.

- *Age two:* Running; walking; galloping; jumping; and swimming with adult help and supervision
- *Age three:* Hopping; climbing; riding a tricycle or bicycle with training wheels and a helmet; and catching, throwing, and kicking a ball
- *Age four:* Skipping, playing tag, sledding, swimming, and completing an obstacle course
- *Age five:* Riding a bicycle while wearing a helmet; somersaulting; rollerblading or ice skating; gymnastics; soccer; and virtual fitness games (such as games for the Wii)

FUN PHYSICAL ACTIVITIES FOR PRESCHOOLERS

Outdoor Activities	Indoor Activities
Games in the yard or park	Duck-duck-goose
Walking the dog together	Follow the leader
Family walks after dinner	Treasure hunt
Freestyle dance	Playing with the dog
Playing catch	Hide-and-seek
Family bike rides	Ring around the rosy
Building a snowman	Simon says
Throwing a Frisbee	Red light, green light
Swimming at a pool or beach	Walking around the shopping mall

Adapted from MyPlate Web site. *www.ChooseMyPlate.gov/Preschoolers /PhysicalActivity.*

Physical Activity Guidelines for Kids in Action

You're probably wondering how your busy child or teen is going to squeeze in 60 minutes a day of physical activity, especially when he or she needs a combination of aerobic, muscle-strengthening, and bone-strengthening activities. As we mentioned before, many physical activities fall under more than one type of activity. This makes it possible for kids to do two or three types of physical activity in one day and it all counts toward their 60-minute daily goal. For example, if your son is on a basketball team and practices with his teammates every day, he is doing vigorous-intensity aerobic activity as well as bone-strengthening activity. If your daughter takes gymnastics lessons, she is not only doing vigorous-intensity aerobic activity but also muscle- and bone-strengthening activity. To fit each type of activity into your child's schedule, follow the Physical Activity Guidelines for

Americans and find activities your child enjoys. Here are two examples of what other kids are doing to meet their goal of 60 or more minutes a day of physical activity. You can check them out in greater detail by going to the Centers for Disease Control and Prevention's online resource Physical Activity for Everyone *(www.cdc.gov/physicalactivity/everyone/getactive/children .html)*.

Harold: A Seven-Year-Old Boy

Harold gets 60 minutes of physical activity each day that is at least moderate intensity. Here's what his week of activity looks like:

- *Monday:* Walks to and from school (20 minutes), plays actively with family (20 minutes), jumps rope (10 minutes), does gymnastics (10 minutes).
- *Tuesday:* Walks to and from school (20 minutes), plays on playground (25 minutes), climbs on playground equipment (15 minutes).
- *Wednesday:* Walks to and from school (20 minutes), plays actively with friends (25 minutes), jumps rope (10 minutes), runs (5 minutes), does sit-ups (2 minutes).
- *Thursday:* Plays actively with family (30 minutes), plays soccer (30 minutes).
- *Friday:* Walks to and from school (20 minutes), plays actively with friends (25 minutes), rides bicycle (15 minutes).
- *Saturday:* Plays on playground (30 minutes), climbs on playground equipment (15 minutes), rides bicycle (15 minutes).
- *Sunday:* Plays on playground (10 minutes), plays soccer (40 minutes), plays tag with family (10 minutes).

Harold also meets the Physical Activity Guidelines for Americans by doing vigorous-intensity aerobic activities, bone-strengthening activities, and muscle-strengthening activities on at least three days of the week:

- *Vigorous-intensity* aerobic activities six times during the week: Jumping rope (Monday and Wednesday), running (Wednesday), soccer (Thursday and Sunday), playing tag (Sunday).
- *Bone-strengthening* activities six times during the week: Jumping rope (Monday and Wednesday), running, (Wednesday), soccer (Thursday and Sunday), playing tag (Sunday).
- *Muscle-strengthening* activities four times during the week: Gymnastics (Monday), climbing on playground equipment (Tuesday and Saturday), sit-ups (Wednesday).

Maria: A 16-Year-Old Girl

Maria gets 60 or more minutes of daily physical activity that is at least moderate intensity. In one week, she participates in the following activities:

- *Monday:* Walks dog (10 minutes), plays basketball (50 minutes).
- *Tuesday:* Walks dog (10 minutes), plays tennis (30 minutes), does sit-ups and push-ups (5 minutes), walks briskly with friends (15 minutes).
- *Wednesday:* Walks dog (10 minutes), plays basketball (50 minutes).
- *Thursday:* Walks dog (10 minutes), plays tennis (30 minutes), does sit-ups and push-ups (5 minutes), plays with children at the park while babysitting (15 minutes).
- *Friday:* Plays Frisbee in park (45 minutes), mows lawn (30 minutes).
- *Saturday:* Goes dancing with friends (60 minutes), does yoga (30 minutes).
- *Sunday:* Hikes (60 minutes).

Maria also meets the Physical Activity Guidelines for Americans by doing vigorous-intensity aerobic activities, bone-strengthening activities, and muscle-strengthening activities on at least three days of the week:

- *Vigorous-intensity* aerobic activities four times during the week: Basketball (Monday and Wednesday), dancing (Saturday), and hiking (Sunday).
- *Bone-strengthening* activities four times during the week: Basketball (Monday and Wednesday), dancing (Saturday), and hiking (Sunday).
- *Muscle-strengthening* activities three times during the week: Sit-ups and push-ups (Tuesday and Thursday), and yoga (Saturday).

Play It Safe

If your child or teen has been glued to a screen and living in a push-button, remote-control world, then you may want him or her to warm up gradually to 60 or more minutes of activity a day. Encourage your kids to increase physical activity in small steps and in ways that they enjoy. A gradual increase in the number of days and the time spent being active will help reduce the risk of injury.

Also, recognize that kids who are overweight may not feel comfortable participating in organized sports. Talk to your child or teen about what types of physical activities he or she would like to try. Some kids may prefer taking lessons rather than playing a sport. Many youth centers, park districts, and YMCAs offer fun physical fitness programs for kids of all ages.

For kids who are currently getting 60 minutes of physical activity every day, be sure to encourage them to continue being active and, if appropriate, increase their activity level. Evidence suggests that being active for more than 60 minutes every day may provide additional health benefits, particularly in terms of achieving and maintaining a healthy weight.

Actively Keeping Track

As a parent, you can help shape your child's or teen's attitudes and behaviors toward physical activity. Since heavy and overweight kids are often reluctant to exercise, it's important to make physical activity part of your *family's* daily routine. To help everyone get started, have each family member aim for at least 60 minutes of physical activity a day and keep track of their progress in a daily log where you note the day, the type of activity, the length of the activity, and who participated. A simple notebook or calendar will work, or you can go online and download the Sample Daily Activity Log from the WeCan! Web site *(WeCan.nhlbi.nih.gov)*. WeCan! (**W**ays to **E**nhance **C**hildren's **A**ctivity & **N**utrition) is a public education outreach program designed to help children ages 8 to 13 stay at a healthy weight through improving food choices, increasing physical activity, and reducing screen time. In addition to the physical activity log, you will find all kinds of other helpful tools on the Web site that you can use to help your family reach a healthy weight.

Physical Activity: Kids Just Want to Have Fun!

The key to getting kids to be more physically active is to focus on the *fun*-damentals—family and fun. As we've noted many times throughout this book, the best way to help kids reach a healthy weight is to make sure the entire family is involved. It's hard for anyone to make changes on their own. Creating family habits around daily physical activity can make it easier for your child or teen to reach and maintain a healthy weight. Also, be sure to factor in fun. Just like kids eat food because it tastes good, the same logic applies to being active. According to a Fitness for Youth survey *(www .fitnessforyouth.umich.edu)*, the two main reasons kids participate in sports and exercise are to have fun and to socialize. Here are several ideas to help you take action and get started with physical activity for a healthy weight lifestyle:

- *Be the family team captain.* Kids look up to their parents as role models. If you make daily physical activity a priority, your child or teen will follow your lead. Kids are more likely to limit TV and computer screen time if you do, and if they have fun family alternatives. And remember, as captain you get to call the plays. Kids will be more likely to listen to your request to "go outside and play!" when you join in.

- *Turn chores into fun activities.* Rake leaves together and take turns jumping in the piles. Shovel snow together and build a snowman or fort. Wash the car and have a water fight. Garden together and see who can pull the most weeds.

- *So you think you can dance?* Gather the family together after dinner and have a dance contest in which everybody takes turns showing off their moves, or make up a family dance routine or skit that you practice a couple evenings a week.

- *Plan an action-packed family adventure.* Spend the weekend bike riding, horseback riding, or hiking together. Plan a family vacation to the beach, canoeing, or camping.

- *Come to the net.* Set up a badminton net in your backyard or at the park. Use it to play badminton, volleyball, or tennis. Let your kids use their imagination and come up with their own games.

- *Dive in.* Spend the afternoon at the local pool, public beach, or water park. Build sand castles, play Marco Polo, and let the kids take turns diving for treasures like dive sticks or pennies.

- *Celebrate special days with live action.* Plan birthday parties, graduations, and family reunions around fun activities like bowling, playing softball, or going to a park or playground. Play active party games such as musical chairs, freeze dance, horseshoes, and relay races.

- *Join a fitness center.* Sign up for a family membership to your local park district, YMCA, or gym. Look for places that offer classes like yoga, basketball, wall climbing, martial arts, and weight lifting.

- *Participate actively in charity events.* Sign the family up for active fundraising events like 5-K runs and walkathons.

- *Walk this way!* Encourage everyone to walk more. Instead of texting friends, walk to their house. Walk to school or the store. Take a family walk after dinner and bring the dog. Get off the bus a stop early and walk the extra few blocks. Go to a forest preserve and walk the trails.

- *Design a family obstacle course.* Have your kids help you set up various stations and be creative in the types of activities at each one. You might try hula hoop, jump rope, push-ups, abdominal crunches, jumping jacks, squats, and marching in place. Set a time and have family members move around to each station and perform the activity for one minute. Increase the time by 30 seconds as the family begins to master each station.
- *Step in time.* Have everyone in the family wear a pedometer (a gadget that counts your steps) and track your movement. Compare steps at the end of the day. Set goals or have contests. Decide together on an award for the most steps in one day or one week.

Healthy Eating, Healthy Weight—You're in Control

◼ *Samantha, her parents, and her brother decided they would all commit to getting fit. They made time to get together and set some goals to get more active. They made a family goal contract to seal the deal:*

> *We, the Davis Family, will work toward the following goal(s) for the next two or three weeks: (1) Remove computers from our bedrooms. (2) Walk our dogs for 15 minutes every night after dinner. (3) Call the park district and enroll in a class. When we have successfully made these a habit, we will reward ourselves with a family bowling night with friends. Signed* Samantha, Peter, Karen, and Tom Davis.

> *They also agreed to keep track of their progress. After a few weeks, they reviewed how they were doing to meet their goals and were very happy with the results. They made bedrooms electronics-free zones and removed all TVs. Samantha moved her computer into the family room so her parents could help her monitor and limit her daily screen time to two hours max. The family also started taking their two dogs for a 15-minute walk*

after dinner every weeknight. Samantha and her friends enrolled in a hip-hop dance class at the park district. On weekends they get together and practice or they play dance video games and work up a sweat from hopping on the control pads. The family decided to reward their hard work by letting Samantha and her brother take a few friends bowling on Saturday night. ■

Kids aren't wired for sitting still all day. Technology may have evolved over the past couple decades to keep them seated at various screens for hours, but their bodies and minds still need plenty of regular physical activity to function well and to stay slim. This is why it is important to follow *Healthy Eating, Healthy Weight Strategy #2: Turn off the tube and move! Limit all screen time to less than two hours a day and be physically active 60 minutes or more a day.*

In this chapter, you have learned a variety of ways that you can help your child or teen turn off the tube and move. As parents, we need to be good role models—remember couch potato parents raise tater tots! Now it's time for your family to come up with some goals that will help everyone step up their daily physical activity. After your family has decided on a few goals, write a contract of your own (*see* the sample form at the end of Chapter 2). As you select goals, have everyone choose activities that are realistic and that they will enjoy.

Here are some examples of possible goals to get your family started:

- Take a 20-minute walk after dinner three nights a week.
- Take a physical activity break during TV commercials by jogging in place, dancing, or doing sit ups.
- Call the local park district or community center and sign up for a class.
- Go on a bike ride on Saturday mornings instead of watching cartoons.
- Limit screen time to two hours each day.
- Pop in a family-friendly exercise DVD in place of a movie or TV program two times a week.

- Each weekend pick one outdoor project that gets everyone moving for one hour, like cleaning the car, raking the leaves, or cleaning out the garage.
- Track your family's progress in a log or on a calendar. At the end of the week, look at what you were able to accomplish. If you were unable to meet a goal, try again or perhaps pick another way to get more active. For example, if your family couldn't enroll in a class at the YMCA, then set up your own 30-minute home fitness class (jumping jacks, walking up and down the stairs, jumping rope, dancing to music) three times a week. Don't be too hard on yourselves. Change takes time! Keep trying and always celebrate your hard work.

5

Healthy Eating, Healthy Weight Strategy #3: Pop the Soda Habit!

■ *Sixteen-year-old Jake Thomas loves having his driver's license. No more riding his bike to the mall or movie theater, now he can cruise over in the car! His dad even lets him drive to high school. Every morning and afternoon, Jake stops by the convenience mart for a biggie cola drink—a 64-ounce soda with unlimited refills for only $1.50. Since Jake never really liked milk, this is a sweet deal. When he was younger, he drank lots of juice and had chocolate milk every once in a while. Now he prefers his cola drinks because the caffeine helps him stay awake. On weekends, he and his friends splurge on mocha coffee drinks topped with whipped cream. In his health class, Jake learned about body mass index and discovered that he was in the obese category for boys his age. As another part of the class project, he used the online MyPlate Food Tracker (www.ChooseMyPlate.gov). He was shocked to see how many calories he was getting each day and that most of them came from beverages. Based on the feedback he got from the MyPlate Food Tracker, Jake decided to try* Healthy Eating, Healthy Weight Strategy #3: Pop the soda habit! Limit sugar-sweetened beverages (such as soda, sport drinks, and fruit punch) to one serving or less a day. ■

Could you imagine letting your child eat 10 chocolate bars at one time or allowing your teen to add 56 teaspoons of sugar to his cereal? Well, if your son or daughter drinks even one 64-ounce soda, like our teenage friend Jake, he or she is unwittingly gulping down the equivalent amount of sugar! And soda is not the only presweetened beverage that kids are drinking these days. They're consuming energy drinks, fruit punch, sweetened coffees and teas, and flavored water—all beverages that contribute too much added sugar and extra calories. This chapter will help you take a hard look at soft drinks and other sugary beverages and the negative role they play in helping kids achieve a healthy weight. It will also provide solutions—beverage choices and sipping strategies that can help your family.

Sugary Drinks: Weighing the Evidence

Are soft drinks, fruit punch, and sport drinks making kids overweight? Although no single beverage may be the cause, drinks with added sugar seem to be a big part of the problem. Over the past few decades, kids have been consuming more calories than they're burning off. About half of the extra calories can be attributed to "liquid calories"—what they're drinking (*see* Liquid Calories Whet Kids' Appetites on page 82)—and this increase in calories just happens to coincide with the rise in childhood obesity. In addition, studies have found that kids who drink the most sugar-sweetened beverages are more likely to be overweight. However, what's really interesting—and hopeful—is that studies have also shown that kids can shed pounds and become a healthier weight if they cut back—or cut out—sugary beverages.

How much of the presweetened stuff are kids drinking? Way too much! In the past decade, soda sipping by kids has popped. On average, kids between the ages of 6 and 11 drink about 15 ounces of soda a day; teens drink even more—about 25 ounces a day. Soft drinks make up the bulk of sweetened beverages kids drink each day; however, compared to years past, they're drinking more of all kinds of sugar-sweetened beverages. Also of note, as kids drink more soft drinks, they drink less milk. In fact, kids today drink more than twice as much soda as compared to milk.

Nobody knows for certain why kids are drinking so many more sugary beverages instead of healthier ones like water or fat-free milk, but portion size may have something to do with it (*see* Chapter 6). In the 1950s, a family-size bottle of cola was 26 ounces. Now a single serving size at fast-food

LIQUID CALORIES WHET KIDS' APPETITES

Did you know that calories from sugary beverages (liquid calories) may be more fattening than calories from food (solid calories)? Our bodies have different systems for monitoring hunger and thirst, and the liquids we drink pass through the stomach more quickly than the foods we eat. As a result, it seems that liquid calories don't trip our built-in satiety system, which helps us feel full. This may explain why many kids can easily drink three or more sugar-sweetened drinks a day. The liquid calories never make them feel full or satisfied so they keep on sipping in addition to eating. However, if kids tried to eat the same amount of solid calories, such as three pieces of chocolate cake, they would probably feel stuffed and eventually put their fork down and stop eating.

restaurants ranges from 12 to 42 ounces, and, as we saw with Jake's story, some convenience marts offer 64 ounces (eight cups)—even if it comes with ice, that's a huge serving. And that's not even counting the free refills!

Drinking such large amounts of soft drinks, fruit drinks, and other beverages with added sugar can be detrimental to your child's or teen's health. Drinks with added sugar provide lots of calories, but they have hardly any of the nutrients kids need to grow (*see* Hey Sugar! on page 84). Too much added sugar may lead to unhealthy weight gain and put kids at risk for tooth decay. Other beverages, such as milk and fruit juice, contain sugar naturally. They too provide calories, but they also contribute nutrients like protein, vitamins, and minerals. Check out the How Much Sugar Is in Your Kid's Cup? chart to find out how much added sugar is in your kid's favorite drink. If that drink is not listed on the chart, check the beverage's Nutrition Facts label for the grams of sugar. Divide that number by four and you will find out how many teaspoons of sugar is in the can, bottle, or carton.

Here are a couple of examples to help you see just how quickly the calories from your kid's cup can lead to an unhealthy weight (keep in mind that 3,500 calories is equal to one pound of body fat):

HOW MUCH SUGAR IS IN YOUR KID'S CUP?

Sweetened Beverage	Calories	Grams of Added Sugar	Teaspoons of Added Sugar
Can of soda (12 ounces)	150	40	10
Soft drink, small (22 ounces)	260	65	16¼
Soft drink, medium (32 ounces)	380	100	25
Soft drink, large (44 ounces)	525	135	33¾
10% juice box (6.75 ounces)	100	23	5¾
Fruit punch (8 ounces)	114	28	8
Lemonade, bottled (20 ounces)	205	55	13¾
Sweetened iced tea (20 ounces)	220	50	12½
Energy drink (8 ounces)	110	27	6¾
Sport drink (20 ounces)	125	35	8¾
Chocolate low-fat milk (8 ounces)	155	16	4

Adapted from Shield J, Mullen MC. *Counseling Overweight and Obese Children and Teens: Health Care Reference and Client Handouts.* Chicago, IL: American Dietetic Association; 2008.

- If a child drank two cups (16 ounces) of fruit punch every day without cutting back on calories from other foods or increasing physical activity, she would gain one pound every two weeks.
- If a teen drank a 64-ounce cola drink every day without cutting back on calories from other foods or increasing physical activity, he would gain one pound every five days.

HEY, SUGAR!

Sugar by any other name is still sugar! *Added sugars* are sugars, syrups, and other caloric sweeteners that are added to foods during processing or preparation, or consumed separately. Added sugars don't include naturally occurring sugars, such as those found in milk or fruits. If you're trying to cut back on added sugars, check food labels for the following ingredients, which are all forms of added sugar:

- Brown sugar
- Cane sugar
- Confectioner's sugar
- Corn sweetener
- Corn syrup
- Dextrose
- Fruit juice concentrate
- Glucose
- High fructose corn syrup
- Honey
- Invert sugar
- Lactose
- Maltose
- Malt syrup
- Molasses
- Raw sugar
- Turbinado sugar
- Sucrose

Beverage Alert!

Many beverages may contain ingredients hazardous to your kid's weight! Let's take a closer look at some of the most popular drinks kids are sipping: soft drinks, energy drinks, sport drinks, fruit drinks, flavored teas, and coffee drinks. To help wean them off, check out the *Think Before You Drink* tips for each type of beverage.

Hard Facts about Soft Drinks

In 2009 sales of carbonated beverages totaled $18.7 billion—that is about $5 billion more than total milk sales! One reason why soft drinks are so popular is the price. Kids learn quickly that they can get more "bang for their buck" by buying a super-size soft drink instead of an 8-ounce carton of low-fat milk. And, let's face it, the variety of types and flavors of soft drinks—regular, diet, with or without caffeine, cola, uncola, and energy drinks—is a temptation trap.

Sweetened Soft Drinks

The main ingredient in sweetened soft drinks is water; they are about 90 percent carbonated water. They provide essentially no key nutrients and are sweetened with either sugar or high-fructose corn syrup, which is a combination of fructose and dextrose (a sugar that comes from corn). There's been a great debate as to whether high-fructose corn syrup may be the reason why obesity rates in the United States have skyrocketed, but there is not enough scientific evidence to say that this sweetener changes metabolism, increases body fat, or boosts appetite. Many companies are removing high-fructose corn syrup from their products, but the key to reaching a healthy weight is to trim calories—cut back on *all* types of added sugar.

Soft drink flavors come from artificial and natural flavors. Acids such as citric acid and phosphoric acid give a tart taste and act as preservatives. Coloring might also be added. Many soft drinks also contain caffeine. While caffeine is not necessarily harmful, it is a stimulant that can affect kids' alertness and sleep patterns; make them feel anxious, jittery, or dizzy; or cause headaches (*see* Caffeine: What's the Buzz? on page 86). Unfortunately, the amount of caffeine is not listed on labels or in the Nutrition Facts, but most caffeine-free soft drinks say so on the label.

If your child or teen drinks sweetened soft drinks, consider these *Think Before You Drink* tips:

- Cut down the quantity over time. Each week, have your kid cut back until he or she reaches the goal of drinking one serving or less a day. And, no, a 64-ounce cup is not a serving! The daily limit should be no more than 8 to 12 ounces, or—better yet—none at all.
- Diet sodas are a better alternative than regular sodas, but water is the best way to quench thirst.
- Serve water or low-fat or fat-free milk at meals instead of soft drinks.

CAFFEINE: WHAT'S THE BUZZ?

For most healthy adults, a moderate amount of caffeine is about 200 to 300 milligrams (mg) a day. A "moderate" amount has not been established for kids, so use common sense. If they're feeling any negative side effects (anxiety, dizziness, headaches, jitteriness) or having trouble sleeping, make sure they cut back or cut out the caffeine.

The following chart lists how much caffeine may be in some of your kid's favorite foods and drinks. For coffee and tea beverages, the caffeine content will vary depending on the brewing methods, plant sources, and brand.

Source	Typical Amount of Caffeine	Range
Brewed coffee (8 ounces)	130 mg	90–150 mg
Cappuccino or latte (8 ounces)	80 mg	60–125 mg
Espresso (single shot; 2 ounces)	80 mg	60–100 mg
Black or green brewed tea (8 ounces)	40 mg	30–60 mg
Flavored iced tea (20 ounces)	25 mg	25–90 mg
Soft drinks (12 ounces)	35 mg	30–60 mg
Energy drinks (8 ounces)	80 mg	50–300 mg
Cocoa beverage (8 ounces)	6 mg	3–32 mg
Chocolate milk (8 ounces)	5 mg	2–7 mg
Milk chocolate (1 ounce)	6 mg	1–15 mg
Dark chocolate, semisweet (1 ounce)	20 mg	5–35 mg
Chocolate syrup (1 ounce)	4 mg	4 mg

Data are from the U.S. Food and Drug Administration.

DIET SOFT DRINKS

Low-calorie, "diet" soft drinks are about 99 percent carbonated water. They contain all the same ingredients as sweetened soft drinks, with one major exception: they don't contain sugar or high fructose corn syrup. Diet soft drinks get their sweet taste from alternative sweeteners, such as aspartame or saccharine. Many parents have concerns about letting their kids consume diet soft drinks, but they seem to be safe. Studies have repeatedly shown that kids and adults can enjoy foods and beverages flavored with alternative sweeteners in moderation and as part of an overall healthy diet. However, compared to fat-free or low-fat milk or 100 percent fruit juice, diet soft drinks offer no nutritional benefits.

Are diet soft drinks an option for your kid? Consider these *Think Before You Drink* tips:

- Once again, choose water over any type of soft drink. It's the perfect calorie-free beverage.
- Kids who drink regular soda can save calories by switching to diet soda.
- Seltzer water with a splash of 100 percent fruit juice is a refreshing, low-calorie fizzy drink.

ENERGY DRINKS

Since they were launched in 1997, energy drinks have become very popular, especially among tweens and teens. There is currently no legal definition of "energy drinks," but, generally speaking, they are super-caffeinated soft drinks that provide added sugar along with other ingredients that may boost energy.

Do kids need energy drinks? According to health experts, the answer is "no." Kids are young and energetic and do not need a boost from a beverage. There are also some safety concerns. For starters, the caffeine content in most energy drinks is very high (up to 300 milligrams per serving) and can exceed the amount in an average 8-ounce cup of coffee (130 milligrams). Also, while the serving size listed on energy drinks is about 8 ounces, large cans of energy drinks are often 23 ounces or more. If a child or teen drank an entire can, they would easily exceed the suggested daily caffeine limit for adults, which is 300 milligrams a day.

Another concern is calories. Although there are a few low-calorie energy drinks, most contain added sugar. For example, one popular energy drink contains 130 calories in an eight-ounce serving, which is more calories than a similar-size soft drink! And as far as added nutrients go, most kids will not benefit from the low levels of vitamins and minerals found in many energy drinks. Energy drinks typically do not add calcium or vitamin D, two nutrients that are missing in action from most kids' cups. Instead you'll find added ingredients such as taurine, guarana, ginseng, and carnitine that allegedly boost energy but have not been proven with research.

If your child or teen consumes energy drinks, consider these *Think Before You Drink* tips:

- Water is the best beverage to keep kids energized!
- Teach kids how to read food labels and do the math. Most energy drinks list the caffeine content per serving. Kids need multiply that amount by the actual number of servings they drink to make sure they do not consume more than 300 milligrams of caffeine a day.
- If kids have an energy drink, make sure it's a low-calorie one.

Know the Score on Sport Drinks

Sport drinks may benefit elite athletes like Lance Armstrong or Serena Williams, but kids should sip water instead. Sport drinks contain up two-thirds the sugar of sodas, and more than three times the sodium (salt). This comes as no surprise if you look at the ingredients list, which typically includes water, high-fructose corn syrup or sucrose, and salt. Many sport drinks also add the electrolyte potassium as well as color and flavor enhancers. The added sugar in sport drinks translates into extra calories and, potentially, unwanted pounds. While it's a good thing to encourage kids to exercise and be active, chances are they will cancel out the calorie-burning benefits if they rehydrate with a sport drinks. Therefore, encourage them to lose the sport drinks.

When talking with your kids about sport drinks, consider *Think Before You Drink* tips:

- Get the winning edge with water—it's the best beverage choice for most active people.
- Dilute sport drinks with an equal volume of water and cut the calories in half.
- Look for lower calorie sport drinks.

Fruit Drinks and Smoothies: The Not So Juicy Details

Don't be fooled by a product name or by the claim, "Contains 20 percent fruit juice." Fruit drinks are basically water with a splash of real fruit juice and lots of added sugar. In fact, according to the 2010 Dietary Guidelines for Americans, fruit drinks were the fourth leading source of added sugar in kids' diets, right behind soda, candy, and sweetened baked goods such as cookies, pies, and cakes. What exactly are fruit drinks? They include fruit punch, fruit "ades" (such as lemonade), and fruit-flavored drinks (such as Kool-Aid)—basically any "fruity" beverage that is not labeled as "juice." By law, only beverages that are 100 percent fruit juice can use the label name "juice" and any beverage that is less than 100 percent fruit juice must list the percentage of the product that is fruit juice and use a descriptive name such as "drink," "punch," or "cocktail." Even though many fruit drinks are fortified with vitamins A and C or other nutrients, they provide more added sugar than anything else. Many kids also order fruit smoothies from juice shops, but they may want to rethink their drink. Most smoothies and blended fruit juice drinks are served in extra-large portions and can be very high in calories.

If your child or teen tends to choose drinks with fruity flavors, consider these *Think Before You Drink* tips:

- Encourage kids to drink water. A squeeze of lemon or lime adds flavor.
- Cut way back or cut out fruit drinks.

- Choose 100 percent fruit juice over fruit drinks.
- Order the smallest size smoothie and make sure it is blended with fat-free milk or yogurt.

Tea and Coffee: Grounds for Concern

Coffee and tea have become popular beverages for tweens and teens. Plain tea and coffee are calorie free, but that is not how kids like to drink them. Here's the scoop on tea and coffee.

Tea

There are basically three types of tea, black, green, and oolong, which come from the *Camellia sinensis* plant. Differences in color and flavor depend on how they are processed. Tea contains caffeine; the longer it is brewed, the more caffeine it has (*see* Caffeine: What's the Buzz? on page 86). Tea has been touted for its health benefits because it contains phytonutrients (iso-flavonoids and polyphenols) that work as antioxidants and may help protect body cells cancer and other health problems. However, most kids drink tea that has been heavily presweetened with more added sugar than you'll find in many soft drinks! This excess sugar really negates any health benefits from tea and often leads to extra calories and pounds.

If your child or teen drinks tea, review these *Think Before You Drink* tips:

- Read the Nutrition Facts label carefully. Bottles of tea often contain 12 to 16 ounces, but the calories listed may be for an 8-ounce serving.
- Look for bottled teas with noncaloric sweeteners.

Coffee

Kids today drink chic coffee drinks such as lattes, cappuccinos, and mochas, often with a shot of caramel, chocolate, or vanilla syrup and topped with whipped cream. These coffee drinks can have more added sugar and fat than a milkshake! Also, many are loaded with caffeine (*see* Caffeine: What's the Buzz? on page 86).

To help your child or teen make healthy choices, review these *Think Before Your Drink* tips regarding coffee:

- Custom order coffee drinks. Request fat-free milk, no (or less) whipped cream, and sugar-free syrup.
- Order the smallest size.
- Encourage kids to go online and check out the calorie content for their favorite coffee drink!

Dear Diary—Tracking Your Kid's Beverage Consumption

If your son or daughter has been drinking large amounts of sweetened beverages, then it will take time to reach the stated goal of *Healthy Eating, Healthy Weight Strategy #3: Pop the soda habit! Limit sugar-sweetened beverages (such as soda, sport drinks, and fruit punch) to one serving or less a day.* Keeping a beverage diary can help kids make progress. Use a small notebook to keep tabs on all beverages. Write down what kids drank, how much, what time, and where. Then go to the MyFood-a-pedia tool *(www .myfoodapedia.gov),* which you can use to analyze the diary page to learn about the calories and food groups in the beverages consumed. Older kids can keep their own drink diaries. Studies have found that simply keeping a diary and being aware of what you're eating or drinking often helps people cut back and reach a healthy weight.

Smart Sippin' Beverages

The best way to implement *Healthy Eating, Healthy Weight Strategy #3: Pop the soda habit! Limit sugar-sweetened beverages (such as soda, sport drinks, and fruit punch) to one serving or less a day* is to teach kids how to be smart sippers.

Hands down, water is the best beverage for kids, followed by fat-free and low-fat milk, and, on occasion and in limited quantities, fruit juice. Let's take a closer look at each of these healthy weight beverages.

Water: Go With the Flow

To help kids cut out sugary beverages, make sure they drink plenty of water. Water is one of the body's most essential nutrients. People may survive six weeks without any food, but they couldn't live more than a week or so without water. That's because water is the cornerstone for all body functions. It's the most abundant substance in the body, accounting for up to 75 percent of body weight. It helps keep body temperature constant at about 98.6 degrees, and it transports nutrients and oxygen to all cells and carries waste products away. Water helps maintain blood volume, and it helps lubricate joints and body tissues such as those in the mouth, eyes, and nose. And water is truly a liquid asset for a healthy weight—it's sugar free, caffeine free, and—most importantly—calorie free.

How Much Water Do Kids Need?

The daily amount of water that a child or teen needs will depend on factors such as age, weight, and gender. Air temperature, humidity, a person's activity level, and his or her overall health affect daily water requirements, too. The Kids' Total Daily Water Requirements chart can help you identify about how many liters of water your child or teen needs each day (one liter is about four cups of liquid). These water recommendations are set for generally healthy kids living in temperate climates; therefore, they might not be a perfect fit for your child or teen.

The amount of water that your child or teen needs each day might seem like a lot, but keep in mind that the recommendations in the chart are for *total* water, which includes water from all sources: drinking water, other beverages, and food. For examples of foods and the amount of water they provide, *see* the chart on page 94. Notice that fruits and vegetables have a much higher water content than other solid foods. Their high water content helps keep the calorie level of fruits and vegetables low while their nutrient level remains high—another perfectly great reason for kids to eat more from these food groups (*see* Chapter 7).

So how do you apply total water recommendations to your kid's day? As a rule of thumb, to get enough water, your child or teen should drink at least six to eight cups of water a day and eat the recommended number of

KIDS' TOTAL DAILY WATER REQUIREMENTS

Age Range	Gender	Total Water (Liters/Day)
4–8 years	Girls and boys	1.3
9–13 years	Girls	2.1
	Boys	2.4
14–18 years	Girls	2.3
	Boys	3.3

Note: Total water includes all water contained in food, beverages, and drinking water.

Data are from Institute of Medicine of the National Academies. Dietary Reference Intakes (DRIs) Tables. Recommended Daily Allowance and Adequate Intake Values: Total Water and Macronutrients. *http://iom.edu/Activities/Nutrition/SummaryDRIs/DRI-Tables.aspx.*

servings of fruits and vegetables every day (*see* Chapters 3 and 7). Also pay special attention to your child's or teen's water consumption when he or she is physically active. Before, during, and after any physical activity, kids need to drink plenty of water, especially in hot weather. The goal is to drink one-half to two cups of water every 15 to 20 minutes while exercising.

Water, Water Everywhere

The message, "Kids need to drink more water," sounds simple, but it can be rather confusing because there are so many types of water you can choose. No need to feel tapped out. Here's some advice to help you come to terms with water.

TAP WATER OR BOTTLED WATER: WHAT ARE THE DIFFERENCES?

Tap water and bottled water are both excellent healthy weight options, and both are safe for everyone in your family to drink because the government carefully regulates them to ensure they are free of contaminants and

THE WATER CONTENT OF SELECTED FOODS

Food	Percent Water by Weight
Lettuce	95%
Watermelon	91%
Broccoli	89%
Milk	89%
Carrot	88%
Apple	86%
Yogurt	85%
Kidney beans, boiled	67%
Whole wheat bread	38%
Raisins	15%
Peanuts	6%
Olive oil	0%

Data are from the U.S. Department of Agriculture, Agriculture Research Service. *www.nal.usda.gov/fnic/foodcomp/search.*

impurities. However, we should note one caveat about the safety of tap water: if you live in an older home or apartment complex, your home may have lead pipes, which could transfer lead to drinking water. In these situations, you can attach a filter to remove impurities to any faucets you use for drinking water.

The differences between tap water and bottled water therefore boil down primarily to taste and price. Some people do not like the taste of their local tap water. Often, they are reacting to the slight aftertaste of chlorine, which is used to clean tap water of impurities and microbial contaminants. Bottled water typically is not chlorinated; it's disinfected in other ways. However, the taste of bottled water varies depending on factors like the

Parents Weigh In: Got Fluoride?

I didn't know that most bottled water is not fluoridated!

—LARRY, DAD OF A SIX-YEAR-OLD BOY

original water source, the use of carbonation, or the mineral content (for more information on types of bottled water, check out the Web site of the International Bottled Water Association: *www.bottledwater.org*). With regard to price, tap water is very inexpensive, costing just pennies a year. In comparison, the price of bottled water adds up quickly. For example, if an eight-ounce (one cup) bottle of water costs $1, and your child drinks eight cups a day, you'll be spending $8 a day and $2,920 a year!

Another consideration in choosing between tap and bottled water is whether it is fluoridated. Some communities fortify their drinking water with fluoride, a mineral that helps strengthen tooth enamel and prevent cavities. Fluoridated tap water should contain 0.7 to 1 parts fluoride per 1 million parts water. Check with your county health department to find out how much fluoride is in your tap water. A few bottled waters are fortified with fluoride, but most are not. Read labels carefully.

Beware of Nutrient-Enhanced Water

Many stores sell hip-looking bottles of water enhanced with vitamins, electrolytes, and other nutrients as well as a range of fancy ingredients. Are they worth the extra cost? Not really. Most nutrient-enhanced waters are basically liquid vitamin supplements plus a little added sugar, which can turn these beverages into a calorie-trap for kids. A single eight-ounce serving of some drinks has about 50 calories, but such beverages may be packaged in a bottle that contains 2½ servings. If kids drink the entire bottle (as most kids do), they could easily drink 125 calories—that's the equivalent to the calories in a can of soda pop. As for the electrolytes in the enhanced water, kids do not really need them unless they are working out vigorously for more than an hour a day. While many nutrient-enhanced waters now come in calorie-free options, kids would be much better off drinking plain-old water and getting their extra nutrients and fluids from foods such as fruits and vegetables.

Water—Sip, Sip Hurray!

If you want your child or teen to be a healthy weight, water works best. Here are some quick and easy tips that will have your kids sipping water instead of a sugary drink:

- *Serve water with meals and snacks.* That way kids are sure to get at least four or five cups of water every day.
- *Keep it cool and make it tasty.* Place a pitcher of water in the refrigerator. Try flavoring the water with a few lemon, lime, or orange slices. Halved strawberries and kiwi also make plain water look and taste irresistible. You could also freeze your kid's favorite fruit juice in ice cube trays and let them add a few colorful and flavorful cubes to their cup of water.
- *Buy wacky water bottles.* For each of your kids, purchase a one-liter, colorful water bottle. Fill it in the morning and let your son or daughter take it to sip on the school bus, in the classroom, and during lunch. Refill the bottle after school and encourage your child or teen to sip throughout the evening, too.
- *Invest in a home water cooler.* Kids enjoy going to the water cooler and pressing the button to get themselves a fresh glass of water. Be sure to pick up some fun cups for them to sip from.
- *Raise seat-belt sippers.* Keep a stash of bottled water in the car and the kids can drink water while you drive. They'll be hydrated and you'll be happy if they spill—water is a lot easier to wipe up than sticky juice or soda.
- *Walk on by and sip.* Whenever kids walk by a water fountain, encourage them to take a drink!
- *Set an example.* The best way to get your kids to drink more water is to drink water yourself! Remember: you are their *Healthy Eating, Healthy Weight* hero!

Moo-re Milk!

Milk is an important beverage for growing kids, but their taste for it has soured. Over the past few decades, there's been a disturbing trend: sugar-sweetened soft drinks have replaced milk as kids' top beverage pick. Girls seem to be drinking less than boys. More than half of boys between the ages of 9 and 18 drink less than the recommended three cups of milk (or milk products) a day, while 90 to 95 percent of girls in the same age group drink less than the recommended amount. The daily milk recommendation for kids ages two to eight is two cups, and many kids are falling short for meeting that, too.

Why Is Milk So Important?

Milk is one of the best sources of calcium and vitamin D—two nutrients that most kids don't come close to getting enough of. Both calcium and vitamin D help kids develop strong bones and teeth. Milk and milk products also seem to play a role in preventing heart disease and hypertension. As for weight loss, milk doesn't seem to prevent childhood obesity, but the type of milk that kids drink can play a big part in determining whether they are at a healthy weight.

Homogenized, pasteurized, fortified—labeling terms like these might make you feel like you need a science degree to pick the right milk for your family (*see* Coming to Terms with Milk on page 98). In fact, the choices are not really so confusing. There are essentially four types of milk: whole milk, reduced-fat (2%) milk, low-fat (1%) milk, and fat-free (skim) milk. All types of milk are created equal in terms of major nutrients such as protein, carbohydrate, vitamins, and minerals. However, when it comes to calories, there's a big "fat" difference. Even though you can't see it, the fat in certain types of milk is unhealthy saturated fat, and milk provides cholesterol, too. Furthermore, since fat is a highly concentrated source of calories, the more fat in the milk, the more calories the milk provides (*see* What's in My Kid's Milk? chart on page 98). Therefore, to ensure our kids are a healthy weight, we need to make sure our kids drink milk *and* make sure that it is low-fat or fat-free milk. Simply switching from whole milk to low-fat or fat-free milk without making any other changes can help kids shed extra pounds without them noticing. Just do the math:

- If your child drinks two cups of whole milk a day and switches to low-fat milk, he would trim 420 calories a week and lose a pound about every eight weeks.
- If your teen drinks three cups of reduced-fat milk and switches to fat-free milk, she would trim 630 calories a week and a pound about every five weeks.

COMING TO TERMS WITH MILK

Confused by those scientific words that appear on milk jugs and cartons? Use these explanations to decipher their meaning.

- *Pasteurized milk*—Pasteurization is a process where milk is heated to destroy microorganisms that can cause spoilage and disease. This process, developed by Louis Pasteur, has been around for centuries and is perfectly safe.
- *Homogenized milk*—Homogenization is a process where the fat particles are broken up and dispersed uniformly so the cream will not rise to the top. Use of this process explains why you can't see the fat in milk.
- *Fortified milk*—Fortification is a process that adds nutrients to a food or beverage that were never originally there. For example, milk doesn't naturally contain vitamins A and D, but these important nutrients are added to it. Soy milk is often fortified with calcium, vitamin A, vitamin D, and riboflavin.

WHAT'S IN MY KID'S MILK?

Based on an eight-ounce serving, here's how the four types of milk stack up in terms of calories, fat, and cholesterol. All types provide equivalent amounts of protein, calcium, and vitamin D.

Type of Milk	Calories	Total Fat	Saturated Fat	Cholesterol
Whole	150	8 grams	4.5 grams	25 mg
Reduced-fat	120	5 grams	3 grams	20 mg
Low-fat	100	2.5 grams	1.5 grams	10 mg
Fat-free	80	0 grams	0 grams	5 mg

Milk Matters

There is a lot of misinformation floating around about milk, which may be contributing to kids' daily milk shortage. Here are the answers to some common questions about milk.

Is My Child Old Enough to Drink Low-Fat or Fat-Free Milk?

Kids of all ages need to drink milk. After a child's second birthday is the perfect time to make the switch to low-fat or fat-free milk.

Is It Okay for Kids to Drink Flavored Milk?

Like plain milk, chocolate milk and other flavored milks provide nutrients such as calcium, vitamin D, phosphorous, protein, and riboflavin. However, in addition to the natural sugar (lactose) in all milk, flavored milks also have added sugar. On average, an eight-ounce serving of low-fat milk contains about four teaspoons of added sugar. To put this in perspective, an equivalent amount of soft drink contains seven teaspoons of added sugar but no healthy nutrients. Flavored milk comes in all different fat versions: whole, reduced-fat, low-fat, and fat-free. Because of the added sugar, all flavored milk will provide more calories than their unflavored counterpart. For example, low-fat chocolate milk has 155 calories, whereas plain low-fat milk has about 120 calories. As they work toward a healthy weight, kids would therefore be better off drinking unflavored milk. On the other hand, an occasional glass of flavored milk would be a better choice than a soft drink or no milk at all.

What If My Child Can't Drink Milk?

Kids diagnosed with a *milk allergy* by a doctor need to avoid drinking milk and eating foods that contain milk. On the other hand, kids diagnosed with *lactose intolerance* may be able to drink milk and eat some dairy products. Kids with lactose intolerance produce too little of the enzyme lactase, an enzyme that the body needs to break down the natural sugar in milk (lactose). Many kids with lactose intolerance can drink up to two glasses of milk a day if the servings are spaced apart (such as one glass in the morning at breakfast and one in the evening with dinner). They also can usually eat dairy foods such as yogurt and cheese, which contain lower amounts of lactose. Finally, there are many varieties of lactose-reduced milk and lactose-free milk available in the supermarket, or kids can take a chewable or swallowable lactase supplement before drinking milk.

If your child or teen has a milk allergy or is lactose intolerant, a registered dietitian (RD) can help you make sure that they're getting enough calcium and vitamin D.

How Does Soy Milk Compare to Cow's Milk?

Soy beverages are made by pressing and then grinding cooked soybeans, and their nutrient content is quite different than cow's milk. Soy milk is lower in protein and riboflavin, has little vitamin A or D naturally, and contains very little calcium. Some soy beverages are fortified with vitamins A and D and riboflavin, and many are fortified with calcium (*see* Coming to Terms with Milk on page 98). If kids are drinking soy milk as a substitute for cow's milk, check the label to make sure the soy milk is fortified with these important nutrients.

Are There Hormones in Milk?

BST, which is short for "bovine somatotropin" (also called "bovine growth hormone" or BHG), is a protein in all cow's milk and beef. It has no effect on humans—like other proteins, it's broken down during digestion.

Small quantities of BST naturally occur in cow's milk. When given as a supplement in small, controlled doses, BST helps cows produce milk efficiently. The normal level of BST in milk itself doesn't change with supplementation because the cow itself uses up the protein. In addition, there's no change in the flavor or nutritional qualities of milk produced from supplemented cows. As always, milk remains an excellent source of calcium, protein, vitamins, and other nutrients.

In 1990 the National Institutes of Health reinforced that BST is safe for humans. In 1993 the U.S. Food and Drug Administration (FDA) approved BST supplementation of cows based on its safety for humans, cows, and the environment.

Milk—Sip, Sip Hurray!

To sum up, kids need to drink milk for good health. For a healthy weight, they need to drink fat-free or low-fat milk. Here are some quick tips help your kids warm up to milk:

- *Lose the fat over time.* Work kids down the milk-fat chain in gradual steps. If they are used to whole milk, switch to reduced-fat milk. After a month or so, switch to low-fat milk. When they are used to that type, step down again to fat-free milk.
- *Milk it at meals.* Serve low-fat or fat-free milk at every meal and snack—that is an easy way to get in three servings a day.
- *Refuel with milk.* When kids are on the go, have them grab a carton or box of low-fat or fat-free milk instead of a soft drink.

Get Juiced!

It's true: 100 percent fruit juice is a nutritious beverage that provides vitamins, minerals, and phytonutrients (*see* Chapters 3 and 7). But drinking too much of it may not be wise for kids trying to reach a healthy weight. Fruit juice is part of the MyPlate fruit group, but fruit juice does not provide the same amount of fiber as whole fruit. Currently, fruit juice accounts for more than half of kids' MyPlate fruit group servings; they're choosing to eat whole fruit only 43 percent of the time. To encourage kids to eat more whole fruit, the American Academy of Pediatrics recommends limiting fruit juice to 4 to 6 ounces a day for kids ages 1 to 6 years. For kids ages 7 to 18 years, limit juice to 8 to 12 ounces a day.

> **Kids Weigh In: Unlimited Juice**
>
> I thought I could drink as much juice as I wanted because it's part of the fruit group.
> —KENDRA, AGE 11

Fruit Juice—Sip, Sip Hurray!

Here are some points to keep in mind regarding fruit juice:

- *Beware of juice overload.* Keep an eye on portion size. Many containers of juice are well over the recommend six- to eight-ounce serving size!
- *Give juice a boost.* Purchase juices fortified with calcium and vitamin C for an added nutrient boost.
- *Be creative and mix flavors.* Combine pineapple juice with carrot juice for a 100 percent fruit and veggie blend.

Healthy Eating, Healthy Weight—You're In Control!

■ *Jake's health class project turned out to be an important wake-up call. He was disgusted to see how much sugar he was guzzling down with his super-size soft drinks and coffee mochas. He also was not happy about the extra weight he had gained. So Jake decided to make some changes and started by filling out the goal contract from his health class book:*

I, Jake Thomas, will work toward the following goal(s) over the next two to three weeks: (1) Switch to the smallest size (22-ounce), low-calorie soda and pass on the refills. (2) Drink water at meals and carry a water bottle in my backpack. (3) Order a latte made with fat-free milk instead of a regular one. When I have successfully made these a habit, I will reward myself by buying five new songs and downloading them to my computer. Signed: Jake Thomas.

In addition to working toward the goals in his contract, Jake kept a drink diary to help him become a smart sipper. He has already started to lose a few pounds. Although he admits it has been hard making the changes, Jake is motivated to continue and talked with his mom and dad about his weight. Since they have a family history of heart disease, they agreed to schedule a check-up with his doctor to make sure he is okay. Jake's mom also agreed to start cooking healthier meals, and his dad will look into joining the YMCA so Jake can exercise more. ■

Nowadays kids are not only eating too many high-calorie, sugary foods, they're drinking them, too! Liquid calories seem to be one of the culprits contributing to the obesity epidemic in this country. Encourage your child or teen to become a smart sipper and follow *Healthy Eating, Healthy Weight Strategy #3: Pop the soda habit! Limit sugar-sweetened beverages (such as soda, sport drinks, and fruit punch) to one serving or less a day.*

Are you ready to complete a family goal contract so your family can become smart sippers? (*See* the sample contract at the end of Chapter 2.) Here are some possible goals to get your family started:

- Cut back to drinking soda pop on the weekends only.
- Bring water bottles to sporting events instead of sport drinks or juice.
- Drink a glass of low-fat or fat-free milk at each meal.
- Order the smallest size soda pop or lemonade when eating out and skip the refills.
- Eat a piece of fruit for breakfast instead of drinking a glass of juice.
- Keep a pitcher of cold water in the fridge at all times (flavor with fresh lemon, lime, or orange wedges).
- Drink no more juice than the recommended daily limit: 4 to 6 ounces (younger kids); 8 to 12 ounces (older kids and adults).
- Switch from whole milk to low-fat milk.

After you set goals and write your family contract, keep a drink diary for each family member. Older kids can keep their own. The information from the diaries will help you complete a tracking record, like the one at the end of Chapter 2, to note your progress. Gather together and check out how everyone is doing with the goals. If you find there are a few setbacks don't get discouraged. Stay positive and support each other.

6

Healthy Eating, Healthy Weight Strategy #4: Practice Portion Control!

■ *Getting six-year-old Stephanie Ramirez to eat has never been a problem. Rather, the challenge has been getting her to cut back. She's the biggest girl in her first grade class. Stephanie eats all her meals and snacks slowly and deliberately—and she always cleans her plate. Most of the time, she begs for seconds. At birthday parties, Stephanie is the last one to leave the table when the pizza or birthday cake is served. When she visits her dad and stepmom on weekends, her favorite activities are going to fast-food restaurants and going out for ice cream. She usually orders a triple-scoop waffle cone with extra candy sprinkles on top.*

One afternoon while Stephanie's mom, Elena, was picking her up from afterschool care, the program director, Tomas, asked to speak with her in private about Stephanie's weight and eating habits. Tomas was concerned that Stephanie seemed to spend more time eating than playing with the other kids. He also said some of the other kids have been saying things to Stephanie about her weight. Elena confessed that she was also worried about Stephanie's weight. Her clothes were so tight around her tummy but the length seemed fine. At Stephanie's last checkup with the pediatrician, Elena and the doctor had talked about Stephanie's weight and the need to make some changes. Elena has been meaning to make some changes, but she is so busy juggling work and getting things done at home. Elena asked

Tomas for suggestions and he encouraged her see a registered dietitian (RD) and try Healthy Eating, Healthy Weight Strategy #4: Practice portion control! Cut food and beverage portions down to the sizes recommended in MyPlate. ■

Over the years, there's been a lot of emphasis on *what* kids should eat—and that is certainly important, especially for health. But portions seem to keep expanding, and therefore kids today need to focus on *how much* they're eating, too. Research has demonstrated that the larger the portion, the more you eat. In fact, eating too much of anything—even healthy foods—will lead to weight gain if calories consumed are not burned off through extra physical activity. Like Stephanie's family, many families are struggling with super-size portions. This chapter will help you learn how to offer kids' portions that are neither too big nor too small, but just right. Learning how to downsize portions can help everyone in the family eat healthier and achieve a healthy weight.

Portions: A Growing Problem

When you were a kid, one thing is for certain: portion sizes were a lot smaller. Over the past few decades, food and drink portions have grown larger—right along with kids' weights. How much larger are portions today? To find out, take the Back to the Future Portion Size Quiz (page 106).

Portion Size Matters

Food and beverage portions have become two, three, four, even five times larger in recent years. What's the big deal? Getting more food, especially when it's low in cost, may seem appealing, but bigger does not mean better. More is not always best. While it may cost the food

---

Parents Weigh In: Cookbook Calorie Creep

I was surprised that even cookbooks are experiencing portion distortion. Years ago, a chocolate chip cookie recipe used to make 100 cookies. Today the exact same recipe makes 60 cookies.

—CAROL, GRANDMOTHER OF 10 KIDS

BACK TO THE FUTURE PORTION SIZE QUIZ

1. Twenty years ago, a bagel was three inches in diameter and had 140 calories. How many calories do you think are in today's bagel?
   - a. 150 calories
   - b. 250 calories
   - c. 350 calories

2. Twenty years ago, a cheeseburger had 333 calories. How many calories do you think are in today's cheeseburger?
   - a. 590 calories
   - b. 620 calories
   - c. 700 calories

3. Twenty years ago, a portion of soda was 6.5 ounces and had 85 calories. How many calories do you think are in today's portion?
   - a. 200 calories
   - b. 250 calories
   - c. 300 calories

4. Twenty years ago, a serving of French fries was 2.4 ounces and had 210 calories. How many calories do you think are in today's portion?
   - a. 590 calories
   - b. 610 calories
   - c. 650 calories

5. Twenty years ago, two slices of pepperoni pizza had 500 calories. How many calories do you think are in two large pizza slices today?
   - a. 850 calories
   - b. 1,000 calories
   - c. 1,200 calories

6. Twenty years ago, a chocolate chip cookie was 1.5-inches in diameter and had 55 calories. How many calories do you think are in today's extra-large chocolate chip cookie?
   - a. 210 calories
   - b. 230 calories
   - c. 275 calories

Answers: 1 c; 2 a; 3 b; 4 b; 5 a; 6 c.

How Your Score Compares

Number of correct answers:

0–2: Uh, oh! Better start paying attention to portion sizes and calories.

3–5: Not bad! Keep paying attention to portion sizes and calories.

6–7: Great! Knowing your portion sizes and calories can help your child or teen reach and maintain a healthy weight.

Adapted from NHLBI Portion Distortion Quiz *(http://hp2010.nhlbihin.net /portion)* and Shield J, Mullen MC. *Counseling Overweight and Obese Children and Teens: Health Care Reference and Client Handouts.* Chicago, IL: American Dietetic Association; 2008.

and restaurant industry only a few extra pennies to scale-up portions, kids pay a hefty price in terms of pounds. Super-size portions are no nutritional bargain. Large portions result in calorie-creep and may lead to an unhealthy weight (*see* Are You Feeding Your Kid Too Much? on page 108). Let's take a look at two primary reasons why portion size matters:

- *I can't believe I ate the whole thing!* A sandwich, a can of soda, a candy bar, a double cheeseburger, a personal pan pizza—it's human nature to eat or drink in single-serve units. No matter how big or how small, most people eat the whole thing. If a small package of potato chips contains three servings, do you think kids will stop after eating just one? In reality, it's much easier (and tempting) to eat the entire package rather than save two servings for later. The result? Instead of eating 150 calories worth of potato chips (one serving), kids eat the entire 450-calorie bag—300 calories more than they anticipated!

- *The more the merrier.* For anyone age five and older, the larger the portion of food plunked down on the plate or poured into a bucket-size cup, the more they eat and drink. How much more? According to studies conducted at Pennsylvania State University, many people eat 30 to 50 percent more when the portions in front of them expand. What's even more shocking, even if we consume more, we don't necessarily feel stuffed. As a result, we don't cut back at other meals and end up going over our daily calorie quota (*see* Appendix A). For example, even if a teenage boy ate an extra-large portion of spaghetti at lunch, chances are he would still eat his usual amount of food at dinner that night. By not compensating for the calorie overload at lunch—either by eating less or exercising more—over time such extra calories can lead to an unhealthy weight. Keep in mind that kids younger than age five do seem to be able to compensate and balance their calories, but, for some reason, most of us lose this ability around age five (*see* Chapter 7).

Portion Size versus Serving Size: What's the Difference?

Portion size and *serving size*—too often these terms are used interchangeably when, in fact, they are not the same. To help your child or teen achieve a

ARE YOU FEEDING YOUR KID TOO MUCH?

Be on the lookout for the following five signs of overfeeding of children and tweens. Your children may have too much on their plates (literally) if:

- They spend lots of time playing with their food rather than eating it all.
- They come to meals and snacks saying, "I'm not hungry!"
- The food portions on their plates are the same as yours.
- They are upset, stressed, tired, or cranky, and you comfort them with food instead of hugs.
- Their clothes are tight in the chest, waist, or rear, even though the length is still fine.

healthy weight, it's important to understand the difference between a "portion" and a "serving." When talking about what kids eat or drink, keep these definitions in mind:

- *Serving size:* A *serving* is a specific amount of food or drink that is defined by common measurements, such as cups, ounces, or tablespoons. Examples include recommended servings from MyPlate (the amount kids *should* eat) and the serving size on a Nutrition Facts label, which is the basis for all the other nutrition information on the label (*see* the following section, Who Determines Serving Size?).
- *Portion size:* A portion is basically the amount of food that happens to end up on the plate. Think of portion size as the actual amount of food kids *choose* to eat at breakfast, lunch, dinner, or a snack. Portions can be bigger or smaller than the recommended serving size.

Who Determines Serving Sizes?

In the United States, there are two main entities that define serving sizes: the U.S. Department of Agriculture (USDA) and the Food and Drug Administration (FDA). The USDA's MyPlate *(www.ChooseMyPlate.gov)* provides *recommended* serving sizes for each of the five food groups and the oil category (*see* Chapter 3). In addition, the FDA, which is responsible for most food product labeling, determines the serving sizes used on the Nutrition Facts panel on packaged foods. In many cases, the serving size listed on the Nutrition Facts label is different from the MyPlate recommended serving size. In fact, many of the MyPlate serving sizes are smaller than those listed on the Nutrition Facts label. However, it is important to be familiar with both types of serving sizes because together they can help you implement *Healthy Eating, Healthy Weight Strategy #4: Practice portion control! Cut food and beverage portions down to the sizes recommended in MyPlate.*

MyPlate Serving Size–Savvy

Since portions have morphed into mega-sizes, kids have grown accustomed to thinking huge quantities of food and beverages are normal. Kids today are clueless about recommended serving sizes that will help them reach and maintain a healthy weight. If kids don't know how much they should be eating, they may be more likely to overeat and gain too much weight. The best way to help kids reach a healthy weight is for everyone in the family to learn how to downsize portions so that they align with the MyPlate recommended serving sizes.

Serving Size Counts

The recommended serving sizes of MyPlate are based on the Dietary Guidelines for Americans and take into consideration the nutrient content as well as the calorie content of specific foods. MyPlate serving sizes are provided for each food group: Grains, Fruits, Vegetables, Dairy, and Protein Foods (*see* MyPlate Recommended Serving Sizes chart). When you visit the My-Plate Web site *(www.ChooseMyPlate.gov),* you can go through each food group and click on photos of the recommended serving sizes for hundreds of different foods.

Note: As we explain in greater deal in Chapter 3, children and teens should stay within their *daily* MyPlate plan for the number of servings they eat from each food group. Therefore, there's no need to eat the exact My-Plate serving size for a food at a particular time. For example, a child whose MyPlate daily plan includes 6 servings (6 ounces) of grains and 5 ounce-equivalents of protein foods could certainly have a sandwich made with two slices of whole wheat bread and 1½ ounces of turkey (2 Grain servings, 1½ Protein Foods servings) at lunch, as long as her meals and snacks for the whole day met (and did not exceed) her daily goals for these food groups.

MYPLATE RECOMMENDED SERVING SIZES

Food Group	Recommended Serving Size	Food Examples
Grains	1 ounce-equivalent	1 slice of bread 1 cup ready-to-eat cereal (except granola) ½ cup cooked rice, pasta, or cooked cereal
Fruits	1 cup	1 cup sliced fruit ½ cup dried fruit 1 piece of whole fruit (about the size of a tennis ball)
Vegetables	1 cup	1 cup raw or cooked vegetables 1 cup vegetable juice 2 cups leafy greens

MYPLATE RECOMMENDED SERVING SIZES
(continued)

Food Group	Recommended Serving Size	Food Examples
Dairy	1 cup	1 cup milk 1 cup yogurt 1½ ounces natural cheese 2 ounces processed cheese
Protein Foods	1 ounce-equivalent	1 ounce meat, poultry, or fish ¼ cup cooked dry beans 1 egg 1 tablespoon peanut butter ½ ounce nuts or seeds

Adapted from MyPlate Web site. *www.ChooseMyPlate.gov.*

MyPlate Portion Distortion

When kids follow the MyPlate recommendations for daily servings, they are well on their way to healthy eating and a healthy weight. Unfortunately, many kids today seem to be suffering from "portion distortion"—the more they're given, the more they will eat. How much are kids overeating? The MyPlate Portion Distortion chart (page 112) illustrates how a typical portion compares to a MyPlate recommended serving. Use this chart to help everyone in your family practice portion control. For example, if your child picked up a bagel at the convenience store, a common portion size would be about four ounces. However, the MyPlate recommended serving size for a bagel is one ounce. Therefore, the entire bagel would count as four MyPlate servings from the Grain group.

MYPLATE PORTION DISTORTION

Food	MyPlate Serving Size	Typical Portion
Bagel	½ bagel: 3 inches in diameter (1 ounce)	1 bagel: 4½ inches in diameter (4 ounces) = **4 MyPlate servings**
Muffin	1 muffin: 2½ inches in diameter (1½ ounces)	1 muffin: 3½ inches in diameter (4½ ounces) = **3 MyPlate servings**
Pancakes	1 pancake: 4 inches in diameter (1½ ounces)	4 pancakes: 5 inches in diameter (9 ounces) = **6 MyPlate servings**
Flour tortilla	1 tortilla: 7 inches in diameter (1 ounce)	1 tortilla: 9 inches in diameter (2 ounces) = **2 MyPlate servings**
Popcorn	2 cups	16 cups (medium movie theater container) = **8 MyPlate servings**
Hamburger bun	½ bun	1 bun = **2 MyPlate servings**
Spaghetti	½ cup (cooked)	2 cups (cooked)= **4 MyPlate servings**
Baked potato	1 small (2⅓ ounces)	1 large (7 ounces) = **3 MyPlate servings**
French fries	½ cup; 10 fries (1 ounce)	1 medium order (4 ounces) = **4 MyPlate servings**
Fried chicken	3 ounces	3 pieces (9 ounces) = **3 MyPlate servings**
Sirloin steak (cooked, trimmed)	3 ounces	12ounces = **4 MyPlate servings**

MYPLATE PORTION DISTORTION *(continued)*

Food	MyPlate Serving Size	Typical Portion
Deli meat sandwich	3 ounces	12 ounces = **4 MyPlate servings**
Fruit juice	1 cup (8 ounces)	20 ounces = **2½ MyPlate servings**
Salad dressing	1 teaspoon	1 ladle (1 ounce) = **6 MyPlate servings**

Adapted from How Much Are You Eating? USDA *Home and Garden Bulletin* No. 267-1, March 2002.

Visualizing Appropriate Portion Sizes

One reason kids may not be eating appropriately sized portions based on the recommended MyPlate servings sizes is that they may not recognize what a reasonable portion looks like. What does one-half cup of pasta look like? What about three ounces of chicken or two tablespoons of peanut butter? The good news is that kids don't need a measuring cup or scale to measure the portions they should eat—instead, they can visualize them by using familiar objects, such as a tennis ball or CD, that are similar in size to recommended serving sizes. Before they eat or drink, they can think of the relevant object and choose a portion that matches its size. *See* the Picture This: How to Visualize Portion Sizes chart (page 114) for some comparisons kids can use. Feel free to come up with your own items to help kids visualize portion sizes.

Portions versus Servings: Dare to Compare?

How do your child's or teen's food and beverage portions compare to the MyPlate recommended serving sizes? Take a look back at the MyPlate Recommended Serving Sizes chart (*see* page 110), and think about the typical portions your child or teen eats at meals or snacks. Are the portions larger

PICTURE THIS: HOW TO VISUALIZE PORTION SIZES

Food	Portion Size	A Portion Is about the Size of
Grains Group		
Bread	1 ounce or 1 regular slice	CD cover
Dry cereal	1 ounce or 1 cup	Baseball
Cooked cereal, rice, or pasta	1 ounce or ½ cup	½ baseball
Pancake or waffle	1 ounce or 1 small (6 inches)	CD
Bagel, hamburger bun	1 ounce or ½ piece	Hockey puck
Cornbread	1 piece	Bar of soap
Fruits Group		
Orange, apple, pear	1 small (2½ inches in diameter)	Tennis ball
Raisins	¼ cup	Golf ball
Vegetables Group		
Baked potato	1 medium	Computer mouse
Vegetables, chopped or salad	1 cup	Baseball
Dairy Group		
Fat-free or low-fat milk or yogurt	1 cup	Baseball
Cheese	1½ ounces natural cheese or 2 ounces processed cheese	9-volt battery
Ice cream	½ cup	½ baseball

PICTURE THIS: HOW TO VISUALIZE PORTION SIZES *(continued)*

Food	Portion Size	A Portion Is about the Size of
Protein Foods Group		
Lean beef or poultry	3 ounces	Deck of cards
Grilled or baked fish	3 ounces	Checkbook
Peanut butter	2 tablespoons	Ping-pong ball
Oils Category		
Tub margarine	1 teaspoon	Standard postage stamp
Oil or salad dressing	1 teaspoon	Standard cap on a 16-ounce water bottle

Adapted from Shield J, Mullen MC. *Counseling Overweight and Obese Children and Teens: Health Care Reference and Client Handouts.* Chicago, IL: American Dietetic Association; 2008.

or smaller than the serving sizes? Remember, even if portion sizes are larger or smaller than the recommended serving sizes, they still may fit into your child's or teen's recommended MyPlate daily eating plan (*see* Chapter 3). For example, a three-ounce portion of fish, poultry, or lean meat is considered a moderate portion size for most older kids; for younger kids, a moderate portion would be about two ounces. The key is to balance all food choices with your child's or teen's calorie needs and physical activity (*see* Chapter 4).

Food Labels: Get the Nutrition Facts

Did you know that almost 40 percent of adults do not read the Nutrition Facts on food labels when they shop for groceries? However, for Healthy

Nutrition Facts

Serving Size 1/2 cup (228g)
Servings Per Container 2

Amount Per Serving

Calories 250   Calories from Fat 110

%Daily Value*

Total Fat 12g	**18**%
Saturated Fat 3g	**15**%
Trans Fat 3g	
Cholesterol 30mg	**10**%
Sodium 470mg	**20**%
Potassium 700mg	**20**%
Total Carbohydrate 31g	**10**%
Dietary Fiber 0g	**0**%
Sugars 5g	
Protein 5g	

Vitamin A 4%	•	Vitamin C 2%
Calcium 20%	•	Iron 4%

* Percent Daily Values are based on a 2,000 calorie diet. Your Daily Values may be higher or lower depending on your calorie needs:

	Calories:	2,000	2,500
Total Fat	Less than	65g	80g
Sat Fat	Less than	20g	25g
Cholesterol	Less than	300mg	300mg
Sodium	Less than	2,400mg	2,400mg
Total Carb		300g	375g
Dietary Fiber		25g	30g

Sample Nutrition Facts for Macaroni and Cheese

Reprinted from WeCan! Web site. Use the Nutrition Facts panel.
www.nhlbi.nih.gov/health/public/heart/obesity/wecan/eat-right/nutrition-facts.htm.

Eating, Healthy Weight kids and families, label reading is essential. Studies have found that people who read and use the Nutrition Facts information tend to eat fewer calories, less sugar, and less fat (particularly saturated "bad" fat). In addition, food labels let you make nutrition-related decisions as you shop, like which container of yogurt has the most calcium and vitamin D.

To understand how to interpret the Nutrition Facts label, let's take a tour of a sample label for macaroni and cheese (above). For more in-depth

information about using the Nutrition Facts label, visit the FDA Web site
(*www.fda.gov/food/labelingnutrition/consumerinformation/ucm078889.htm*).

Start with Servings

When you look at the Nutrition Facts label, start with the serving information. Everything you read on the rest of the label is based on one serving.
There are two parts to the serving information:

- *Serving size* tells you the recommended size for one serving. Serving sizes are listed in common household measures (such as cups,
  ounces, or tablespoons) and in grams; the sizes are standardized to
  make it easier for you to compare similar foods. The serving size
  for the macaroni and cheese is one cup or 228 grams.
- *Servings per container* shows how many recommended servings are
  in the entire package. If your child ate the entire package of macaroni and cheese, he or she would eat two servings (two cups).

Check Calories

The calories section of the Nutrition Facts label can help you manage your
child's or teen's weight. Calories are shown for one serving. For example,
one serving of macaroni and cheese has 250 calories. Remember: the number of servings your child eats determines the actual number of calories he
or she consumes. If your child eats a package of macaroni and cheese (two
cups), that's 500 calories.

Limit These Nutrients

The first five nutrients on the Nutrition Facts label are total fat, saturated
fat, *trans* fat, cholesterol, and sodium. Most kids and adults eat enough or
even too much of these nutrients. Too much fat, saturated fat, *trans* fat,
cholesterol, and sodium may increase one's risk of certain chronic diseases,
like heart disease, some cancers, or high blood pressure (*see* What's Shaking
with Sodium? on page 118). For healthy eating and a healthy weight, kids
should eat as little as possible of these nutrients.

WHAT'S SHAKING WITH SODIUM?

People who eat a diet high in sodium (salt) are at increased risk for high blood pressure, heart disease. and stroke. Early stages of health problems related to blood pressure begin during childhood, so both children and adults should cut back on sodium, working *gradually* toward a goal of 1,500 mg of sodium (or less) per day. That's about two-thirds of a teaspoon of table salt.

Here are a few ways you can help your family shake the salt habit:

- Prepare foods with less, and eventually no, salt. Your taste for salt will gradually decrease over time. Remember: when you cook at home, *you* control the ingredients (*see* Chapter 10).
- Flavor foods with other herbs and spices instead of salt.
- Check food labels for terms like "low sodium" or "sodium free."

Get Enough of These Nutrients

Most kids don't get enough of the nutrients listed toward the bottom of the Nutrition Facts label: dietary fiber, vitamin A, vitamin C, calcium, and iron. Eating enough of these nutrients can improve health and may reduce the risk of some diseases and conditions. For example, calcium helps kids grow and keeps bones strong; dietary fiber promotes healthy bowel function and may play a role in reducing the risk of heart disease. You can use the Nutrition Facts label to make sure kids are getting enough of these nutrients.

Keep an Eye on Percentages

At the far right of the Nutrition Facts label are percentages called % Daily Value (%DV). The %DVs can help you determine whether a serving of food is high or low in a nutrient. Here's how to interpret %DV:

- **Low** amount of the nutrient = 5%DV or less
- **High** amount of the nutrient = 20%DV or more

A couple of notes: First, some nutrients (such as *trans* fat) do not have %DV. Second, the %DV column doesn't add up vertically to 100 percent. Instead, the %DV for each nutrient is based on what would be 100 percent of the daily requirements for that nutrient for people who need to eat 2,000 calories a day. However, you can still use the %DVs as a frame of reference regardless of your kid's daily calorie goal. (To learn your kid's calorie needs, *see* Chapter 3 and Appendix A).

Let's use %DVs from our sample label to see how the key nutrients in the macaroni and cheese stack up. On the positive side: this product is high in calcium and potassium (20%DV for each). On the negative side, this food is low in dietary fiber (0%DV), vitamin A (4%DV), vitamin C (2%DV), and iron (4%DV), and it's high in sodium (20%DV).

Make your kids' calories count. To decide whether a food is worth eating, look at the calories and the amounts of healthy and unhealthy nutrients on the label. For the macaroni and cheese product, the negatives outweigh the positives, so you may want to choose another brand. Alternatively, you could buy this brand and balance any missing healthy nutrients with other foods that provide them at other meals throughout the day.

Take Note of the Footnote

The footnote at the bottom of the Nutrition Facts label shows recommended dietary advice for people based on either a 2,000 calorie or 2,500 calorie diet. It's a good general reminder about how everyone can eat healthier. (Labels on smaller packages may omit this note.)

What Else Is on a Food Label?

In addition to the Nutrition Facts, here are some other important aspects of the food label you'll want to check out. Keep in mind that all information on food labels must meet strict government standards and be approved before it can appear on the label.

Nutrient Content Claims, Health Claims, and Structure-Function Claims

A *nutrient content claim* is an FDA-approved word or phrase on a food package related to the nutritional value of the food, such as "low calorie" or "fat free." The following nutrient content claims can help you easily find foods that will help your child or teen reach a healthy weight. Because the FDA oversees the definitions of nutrient content claims, a particular claim will mean the same thing for every product that uses it.

- *Low calorie:* 40 calories or less per serving
- *Reduced-calorie:* At least 25 percent fewer calories per serving when compared with the original food
- *Light* or *lite:* One-third fewer calories or 50 percent less fat per serving; if more than half the calories are from fat, fat content must be reduced by 50 percent
- *Sugar-free:* Less than one-half gram sugar per serving
- *Reduced-sugar:* At least 25 percent less sugar per serving when compared with the original food
- *Fat-free:* Less than one-half gram fat per serving
- *Low-fat:* Three grams of fat or less per serving
- *Reduced-fat:* At least 25 percent less fat when compared with the original food

A *health claim* describes the potential health benefits of a food, nutrient, or food substance to reduce the risk of a chronic disease or condition, such as cancer, coronary heart disease, or hypertension. Listing this information is optional, and many foods that meet the criteria don't carry the health claim on their labels. All health claims must be supported by scientific evidence and are strictly regulated by the FDA. Examples of health claims that have FDA approval to appear on food labels include:

- *Calcium* and osteoporosis
- *Sodium* and hypertension
- *Dietary fat* and cancer
- *Saturated fat and cholesterol* and the risk of coronary heart disease
- *Fiber-containing grain products, fruits, and vegetables* and cancer

A *structure/function claim* describes how a nutrient or a food substance may affect health. Some examples include: "helps maintain bone health" or "supports a healthy immune system." These claims can't suggest any link to lowered risk for disease. Unlike health claims, structure/function claims do not need FDA approval or review, and they have no specific standards that regulate the wording. However, they still must be truthful and not misleading.

INGREDIENTS LIST

The *ingredients list* on a packaged food gives an overview of the "recipe." By regulation, any food made with more than one ingredient must carry an ingredient list on the label. Food manufacturers must list all ingredients in descending order by weight, which means ingredients are listed from most to least. Take a look at the ingredients list for the macaroni and cheese product we've been using as a label-reading example. Enriched macaroni product is the first ingredient, which means the product contains more macaroni by weight than anything else. Reading the ingredients can help you select products with the least amount of added sugars, solid fats, and sodium while choosing products with more whole grains, dietary fiber, and other important nutrients.

SAMPLE INGREDIENTS LIST FOR MACARONI AND CHEESE

INGREDIENTS: Enriched Macaroni Product (Wheat Flour, Niacin, Ferrous Sulfate [Iron], Thiamin Hydrochloride [Vitamin B1], Riboflavin [Vitamin B2], Folic Acid); Cheese Sauce Mix (Whey, Milkfat, Milk Protein Concentrate, Salt, Sodium Tripolyphosphate, Contains Less than 2% of Citric Acid, Lactic Acid, Sodium Phosphate, Calcium Phosphate, Milk, Yellow 5, Yellow 6, Enzymes, Cheese Culture).

What If There Is No Label?

Nutrition Facts and the ingredients list appear on almost every packaged food in the food market. Labels are not legally required on fresh fruits and vegetables, meat, poultry, and seafood, but these foods may be labeled voluntarily with nutrition information, either on the package or on a poster or a pamphlet displayed nearby. If you don't find this information in your supermarket, ask the store manager to start providing it or check the product's Web site. In addition, many restaurants offer nutrition information either on their menu or on their Web sites (*see* Chapter 8).

How to Keep Track of Portions

To help kids follow *Healthy Eating, Healthy Weight Strategy #4: Practice portion control! Cut food and beverage portions down to the sizes recommended in MyPlate,* have them keep a food diary. Studies have found that many people automatically cut back their food portions when they keep track of what they are eating. Keeping a food diary tends to be an eye-opening experience that helps everyone discover:

- Which foods may be contributing the most calories
- How often, when, and where kids consume these foods
- Which situations trigger kids to eat

There are many ways to keep a food diary. You can simply use pen and paper to note what your child eats for a few days. Record the foods and drinks consumed, as well as the time, location, and amount (ounces, cups, tablespoons, teaspoons, and so on). Teens can keep their own written records. Another option is the online MyPlate Tracker *(www .ChooseMyPlate.gov),* which we discussed in Chapter 3. Tweens and teens who love to use their cellphones may like to use a food tracking app—many are free of charge and can be good tools when kids use them daily.

At least once a week, review and discuss the food diary with your child or teen. Based on the results, help your kid pinpoint changes he or she could make to reduce portion sizes.

How To Cut Portions Down to Size

In addition to using MyPlate, reading food labels, and keeping a food diary, here are some other tips that will help kids following *Healthy Eating, Healthy Weight Strategy #4: Practice Portion Control! Cut food and beverage portions down to the sizes recommended in MyPlate:*

- *Solve the portion puzzle.* Before dishing up plates or filling cups, weigh and measure portions to make sure you know how they compare to the recommended MyPlate serving sizes. Better yet, let kids do the measuring. They will learn what a portion should look like *and* brush up on their science and math skills!

- *Know your dishware limits.* Premeasure your cups, glasses, and bowls by filling them with water and then pouring that water in into a measuring cup to check the volume. That way you'll know how much your dishes hold without having to measure the food portions.

- *Downsize dishes.* Save large dinner plates for special occasions. Use a smaller salad plate to serve meals and serve snacks like ice cream, pudding, and nuts in small bowls or ramekins. Studies have found that smaller dishes trick our brains into thinking we are eating more food because a smaller portion looks large in a little dish.

> ### Kids Weigh In: Bag It!
>
> It's hard to resist eating the whole bag of microwave popcorn. So now I pop it and put it into a small bowl. I share the extra with my brother and sister.
>
> —ERIC, AGE 11

- *Skip seconds—except for fruits and veggies!* When eating at home, dish up appropriate portions on individual plates and place the plates around the table, leaving the serving dishes out of reach. There is one exception to this rule: fruits and vegetables. Keep a large bowl of vegetables and fruit on the table and let kids have seconds of these (*see* Chapter 7).

- *Encourage kids to eat slowly.* After we start eating, it takes about 20 minutes for the stomach to signal to the brain that it's full. Teach kids to put their fork down between bites and alternate with sips of water or fat-free milk. For younger kids, cut up only a few bites at a time and let them ask for more.

- *Out of sight, out of mind.* Make your home a portion-friendly zone. Since kids tend to eat more when they have easy access to food, try replacing the candy dish with a fruit bowl. Move healthier foods like sliced vegetables, fat-free yogurt, and fresh berries to the front of the refrigerator while storing high-fat and sugar-added goodies like chips or cookies on higher shelves and out of immediate sight. Better yet, keep these foods out of the house. You can go out to enjoy them once in awhile as a family treat.

- *Put away the bag.* Make sure kids always eat foods from a plate or bowl and never straight out of a large bag or carton. This helps prevent mindless munching, which often leads to eating much more than one serving.

- *Divide and conquer.* Studies have confirmed that the larger the package, the more people eat from it. To help curtail overeating, divide the contents of one large box or bag of a food into several smaller containers, or purchase single-serve or bite-size packages to help pare down portion sizes.

- *Split meals or dessert.* Save money and calories when eating out by sharing entrées or dessert. Restaurant portion sizes are so large that they often are enough to feed at least two people, especially younger kids (*see* Chapter 10).

- *Keep tools on hand to help end eating.* Having a pack of sugar-free gum or mints on hand may help kids resist the urge to "have just one more bite," snack mindlessly, or eat when they are not hungry.

Healthy Eating, Healthy Weight—You're In Control!

■ *Stephanie's parents and stepparents agreed to meet with a registered dietitian (RD) named Carla. She helped them realize that Stephanie was eating too much for a child her age. Almost all of her portions were twice the serving sizes recommended in MyPlate! Carla recommended that the family fill out a family*

*goal contract, which could help them remember to work togeth-
er as a team. They agreed and wrote:*

> *We, Stephanie Ramirez and family, will work toward
> the following goal(s) over the next one or two weeks:
> (1) Measure food at meals to learn about the "right-size"
> portions. (2) Offer fruits and vegetables for seconds at
> meals. (3) Limit fast food to once every other weekend.
> (4) Order a small ice cream cone with only one scoop in-
> stead of the large one. When we have successfully made
> these a habit, we will reward ourselves by buying Wii Fit
> Dance. Signed: Stephanie Ramirez and family.*

*Stephanie and her dad made plans to replace their weekend
fast-food rituals with home-cooked meals followed by a fun, active outing like a trip to the park or a family bike ride. The adults
learned how to read Nutrition Facts labels when shopping and
they now try to keep their kitchens full of healthier foods.* ■

When working on *Healthy Eating, Healthy Weight Strategy #4: Practice
portion control!*, practice and consistency are key. Like Stephanie's family,
filling out a family goal contract will help ensure everyone is on the same
page. So gather everyone around the table to set a few portion control goals
and make your family contract (*see* the form at the end of Chapter 2). Here
are some examples of possible goals to get you started:

- Dish up meals from the stove instead of serving them family-style
  with the bowls on the table.
- Have your family measure portions for one week, using the
  MyPlate Recommended Serving Size chart as a guide.
- Put snacks into snack-size baggies in portions consistent with
  MyPlate recommended serving sizes.
- Offer vegetables and fruits for seconds, instead of another serving
  of rice or pasta.
- Split the main dish when eating out or order the lunch-size
  portion.

Monitor your progress by completing and reviewing a tracking form like the one shown at the end of Chapter 2. Remember to reward your successes by dishing up a serving of family fun time, such as taking a long hike in the country.

7

Healthy Eating, Healthy Weight Strategy #5: Fill Up on Fruits and Veggies!

◼ *Three-year-old Mario Valentine is such a picky eater, refusing everything except whole milk, fruit drinks, and a limited repertoire of foods that excludes fresh fruits and vegetables. He seems to have no trouble eating at daycare, but the dinner table has turned into a battlefield! His parents have tried forcing him to eat, giving time outs for not eating, and offering food bribes—if you eat your peas, you can have dessert—but nothing seems to work. Tired from working full time and fighting with Mario, they have given in and prepare only the foods he will eat: chicken nuggets, macaroni and cheese, and pizza. They're hoping it's just a stage. After all, Mario used to be a good eater before his mom went back to work full time. At Mario's recent check-up, his pediatrician asked Mario's mom to talk with Donna, the clinic's registered dietitian (RD), because Mario had gained too much weight over the past year. His mom was shocked! How could a picky eater possibly gain too much weight? Donna recommended that Mario and his family try* Healthy Eating, Healthy Weight Strategy #5: Fill up on fruits and veggies! Eat plenty of servings of fruits and vegetables every day. ◼

Kids know the mantra: eat more fruits and vegetables—they're good for you! Unfortunately, they're doing just the opposite—they're eating fewer. On average, kids eat a combined total of one cup of fruits and vegetables a day—well below the recommended amount. If, like Mario's parents, you're tired of fighting the fruit and veggie battle, don't surrender yet. Research shows that kids who eat fruits and vegetables are more likely to be a healthy weight. This chapter will help you make sure your child or teen is eating their daily fruit and veggie quota. You'll learn how many fruits and vegetables kids really need to eat, how to pick the best produce, and how to get kids to love eating fruits and veggies.

Fruits and Vegetables—Good for Health *and* Weight

Why do kids need to eat generous amount of fruits and vegetables? For starters, fruits and veggies provide a cornucopia of nutrients, such as vitamin A, vitamin C, most of the B vitamins, and minerals like potassium, iron, and magnesium. Certain vegetables such as legumes (dried beans, peas, and lentils) also provide protein. All of these nutrients help kids grow properly and stay healthy. In addition, fruits and vegetables contain more than 2,000 types of *phytonutrients*—natural compounds (including plant pigments) that offer health benefits ranging from keeping eyes healthy to possibly warding off cancer and heart disease (*see* Color Kids' Worlds).

Although the benefits of vitamins, minerals, and phytonutrients are reason enough to give fruits and vegetables a prominent place on your kids' plates, these wonder foods also play an important role in weight control. Because most fruits and vegetables contain a lot of water and dietary fiber, they are filling and satisfying—which means kids are less likely to overeat (*see* Chapter 3). They are also naturally free of added sugars and solid fat, and most are "nutrient dense"—that is, they provide a large amount of nutrients for a minimal amount of calories. For these reasons, the *more* fruits and vegetables kids eat, the *more likely* they are to be a healthy weight. Are you interested in seeing how this works? Check out the Fruit and Veggie Calorie Trade-Offs chart (page 130) to see how picking fruits and vegetables instead of higher calorie foods with solid fat and added sugar can help kids reach a healthy weight and meet their daily produce requirements.

COLOR KIDS' WORLDS

Put a rainbow on your kids' plates! Different colors of fruits and vegetables provide different phytonutrients.

Color	Phytonutrients	Potential Health Benefits
Green (*Fruits:* apples, grapes, honeydew, kiwi, and lime; *vegetables:* artichoke, asparagus, avocado, broccoli, green beans, green peppers, and leafy greens such as spinach)	Chlorophyll Lutein Zeaxantinin Beta carotene	May help promote healthy vision and reduce cancer risks
Yellow and orange (*Fruits:* apricots, cantaloupe, grapefruit, mangos, papaya, peaches, and pineapple; *vegetables:* carrots, yellow peppers, yellow corn, and sweet potatoes)	Beta carotene Zeaxantinin	May promote healthy vision and immunity and reduce the risk of some cancers
Purple and blue (*Fruits:* blackberries, blueberries, plums, and raisins; *vegetables:* eggplant, purple cabbage, and purple-fleshed potatoes)	Anthocyanidins	May help with memory and reduce cancer risks
Red (*Fruits:* cherries, cranberries, pomegranate, red/pink grapefruit, red grapes, and watermelon; *vegetables:* beets, red onions, red peppers, red potatoes, rhubarb, and tomatoes)	Lycopene Anthocyanins	May help maintain a healthy heart, vision, and immunity and reduce cancer risks

(continued)

COLOR KIDS' WORLDS (continued)

Color	Phytonutrients	Potential Health Benefits
White, tan, and brown (*Fruits:* banana, brown pears, dates, and white peaches; *vegetables:* cauliflower, mushrooms, onions, parsnips, turnips, white-fleshed potatoes, and white corn)	Flavonols	May promote heart health and reduce cancer risks

FRUIT AND VEGGIE CALORIE TRADE-OFFS

Swap Out	Swap In	Save
1 cup potato chips (107 calories)	12 baby carrots (42 calories)	65 calories
1 large oatmeal raisin cookie (118 calories)	¼ cup raisins (42 calories)	76 calories
1 cup orange drink (119 calories)	1 large orange (62 calories)	57 calories
1 cup corn chips (237 calories)	1 small corn on the cob (88 calories)	149 calories
2-ounce candy bar (237 calories)	1 small banana (90 calories)	147 calories
	Daily Totals:	
Fruit servings = 0 cups Vegetable servings = ¼ cup	Fruit servings = 2¼ cups Vegetable servings = 2 cups	494 calories saved!

Fruits and Veggies: Know Your Kid's Number

Why won't kids eat more fruits and veggies? One reason crops up: quantity. Both kids and parents seem to have unrealistic expectations about what it means to eat "more" fruits and vegetables. Kids don't know *how much* they should be eating, and neither do their parents.

How Many Fruits and Veggies Do Kids Need Each Day?

Kids need to eat different amounts of fruits and vegetables depending on their age, gender, and calorie needs. If you already know your child's or teen's daily calorie needs, you can use the Fruit and Veggie Cups for Kids chart we've provided to determine how many cups of fruits and vegetables your son or daughter needs each day. If you don't know your kid's calorie targets, go to the MyPlate Web site *(www.ChooseMyPlate.gov)* and print a personalized MyPlate daily food plan (*see* Chapter 3 for more information

FRUIT AND VEGGIE CUPS FOR KIDS: DAILY GOALS

	1,000 Calories/ Day	1,200 Calories/ Day	1,400 Calories/ Day	1,600 Calories/ Day	1,800 Calories/ Day
Fruits	1 cup	1 cup	1½ cups	1½ cups	1½ cups
Vegetables	1 cup	1½ cups	1½ cups	2 cups	2½ cups

	2,000 Calories/ Day	2,200 Calories/ Day	2,400 Calories/ Day	2,600 Calories/ Day	2,800 Calories/ Day
Fruits	2 cups	2 cups	2 cups	2 cups	2½ cups
Vegetables	2½ cups	3 cups	3 cups	3½ cups	3½ cups

Adapted from Dietary Guidelines for Americans 2010. Appendix 7. *www.cnpp.usda.gov/DietaryGuidelines.htm.*

about MyPlate, which puts the daily nutrition recommendations from the U.S. government's Dietary Guidelines for Americans into action).

Let's use the chart to find out how many cups of fruits and vegetables our picky eater Mario should be eating each day. Mario is three years old and needs about 1,000 calories a day, so he needs to eat one cup of fruit and one cup of vegetables every day.

What Counts as a Fruit or Vegetable Serving?

Now that you know how many cups of produce your child or teen should eat each day, you may be wondering: What does one cup or one-half cup look like? The Counting Cups of Fruits and Veggies chart lists a few food examples to help you visualize the size (*see* Chapter 6 for more information about visualizing portion sizes). **Note:** 100 percent juice can count toward your kid's daily goal for fruit or vegetables (eight ounces of juice equals one cup), but juice does not provide as much fiber as the "whole" version of the fruit or vegetable. Therefore, kids should focus on eating rather than sipping their daily produce servings (*see* Chapter 3).

Rotate Veggies!

Unlike fruits, the nutrient composition of vegetables varies quite a bit. Some have more protein, others more starch. For this reason, MyPlate (*www.ChooseMyPlate.gov*) classifies all fresh, frozen, and canned vegetables (cooked or raw) into five subcategories based on their main nutrient contribution (*see* Chapter 3). Here are some examples of vegetables in each category:

- *Dark-green vegetables*—broccoli; spinach; romaine lettuce; and collard, turnip, and mustard greens
- *Red/orange vegetables*—tomatoes, red peppers, carrots, sweet potatoes, winter squash, and pumpkin
- *Dry beans and peas (legumes)*—kidney beans, lentils, chickpeas, and pinto beans
- *Starchy vegetables*—white potatoes, corn, and green peas
- *Other vegetables*—iceberg lettuce, green beans, and onions

COUNTING CUPS OF FRUITS AND VEGGIES

	1 Cup Equals	½ Cup Equals
Fruits	1 small apple	1 snack container of applesauce (4 ounces)
	1 small wedge watermelon	½ medium grapefruit
	1 medium pear	1 medium cantaloupe wedge
	1 medium grapefruit	1 large plum
	1 large banana	4 large strawberries
	1 large orange	16 grapes
	2 large or 3 medium plums	1 small box raisins (¼ cup)
	8 large strawberries	
Vegetables	1 medium potato	5 broccoli florets
	1 large bell pepper	6 baby carrots
	1 large sweet potato	½ medium potato
	1 large ear of corn	½ large sweet potato
	12 baby carrots	
	2 medium carrots	
	1 cup cooked or 2 cups raw greens (spinach, collards, mustard greens, or turnip greens)	

Because it's important for kids (and adults!) to eat veggies from all the vegetable subcategories, MyPlate offers a *weekly* vegetable rotation schedule (*see* chart on page 134), which is based on daily calorie needs. Use the schedule as a guideline to help your son or daughter pick a wide variety of veggies each week. It can also help you plan weekly menus that vary your kid's veggies. If the chart seems too complex, stick with this rule of thumb: offer a different colored veggie each day.

WEEKLY VEGGIE ROTATION SCHEDULE

	1,000 Calories/Day	1,200 Calories/Day	1,400 Calories/Day	1,600 Calories/Day	1,800 Calories/Day
Dark-green vegetables	½ cup/week	1 cup/week	1 cup/week	1½ cups/week	1½ cups/week
Red and orange vegetables	2½ cups/week	3 cups/week	3 cups/week	4 cups/week	5½ cups/week
Beans and peas (legumes)	½ cup/week	½ cup/week	½ cup/week	1 cup/week	1½ cups/week
Starchy vegetables	2 cups/week	3½ cups/week	3½ cups/week	4 cups/week	5 cups/week
Other vegetables	1½ cups/week	2½ cups/week	2½ cups/week	3½ cups/week	4 cups/week

	2,000 Calories/Day	2,200 Calories/Day	2,400 Calories/Day	2,600 Calories/Day	2,800 Calories/Day
Dark-green vegetables	1½ cups/week	2 cups/week	2 cups/week	2½ cups/week	2½ cups/week
Red and orange vegetables	5½ cups/week	6 cups/week	6 cups/week	7 cups/week	7 cups/week
Beans and peas (legumes)	1½ cups/week	2 cups/week	2 cups/weeks	2½ cups/week	2½ cups/week
Starchy vegetables	5 cups/week	6 cups/week	6 cups/week	7 cups/week	7 cups/week
Other vegetables	4 cups/week	5 cups/week	5 cups/week	5½ cups/week	5½ cups/week

Adapted from Dietary Guidelines for Americans 2010. Appendix 7. *www.cnpp.usda.gov/DietaryGuidelines.htm.*

Fruit and Veggie Planner

Once you and your kids know how many fruits and veggies they need to eat each day, the next step is getting kids to eat them. A great way for kids to reach their fruit and veggie goals is to encourage them to keep track on a monthly calendar. Look for one with lots of blank space below the dates. Younger kids can draw or color in pictures of the fruits and vegetables they ate each day, and older kids can simply write down the names and how much. Take time at the end of each week to talk with your kids about what their calendar shows. Discuss the types of fruits and vegetable eaten, the nutrients they supply, and how they tasted. Also talk about other fruits or vegetables your child or teen would like to add to the shopping list to try next week.

Produce: Picking the Best Options

When selecting and preparing fruits and vegetables, taste and nutrition are, of course, important. However, as the flurry of media attention regarding pesticides and produce recalls demonstrates, food safety is also a growing concern. Here are some pointers for picking fruits and vegetables that are nutritious, safe, *and* delicious.

Fresh, Frozen, or Canned—What's the Difference?

No matter what form they take—fresh, frozen, canned, or dried—most fruits and vegetables are *Go for It* foods that kids can enjoy any time (*see* Chapter 3 for more information on the concept of *Go for It* foods). All of them count toward your child's or teen's daily fruit and vegetable goals. Here are some selection tips.

FRESH PRODUCE

Fresh produce is always nutritious. Just make sure you pick fruits and vegetables that are free of bruises or cuts—bacteria can get in and cause spoilage. Also, purchase fruits that are ripe and at their flavor peak. Review the Selecting and Storing Fresh Produce chart (page 136) for more tips. A good online source for additional information and videos about how to shop for, store, and prepare fresh produce is the Fruits and Veggies More Matters Web site *(www.fruitsandveggiesmorematters.org)*.

SELECTING AND STORING FRESH PRODUCE

	Selection Tips	Storage Tips
Fruits		
Apple	Choose firm, shiny, smooth-skinned apples with stems still attached. They should smell fresh, not musty.	Refrigerate in a plastic bag away from strong odors. Use within 3 weeks.
Pear	Choose firm fruit, then apply gentle pressure to the stem end of the pear with your thumb to test ripeness. When it yields to pressure, it's ready.	Store unripe pears in a bag at room temperature. Refrigerate ripe pears.
Mango	Choose slightly firm mangos with a sweet aroma. Avoid those with sap on their skin.	Store at room temperature for 1–2 days. Refrigerate peeled, cut mangos.
Watermelon	Choose symmetrical watermelons with dried stems and yellow undersides. They should be heavy for their size.	Store whole watermelons at room temperature. Refrigerate slices or pieces in airtight containers for use within 5 days.
Vegetables		
Acorn squash	Choose acorn squashes that are dull and heavy for their size.	Store in a cool, dry area away from extreme temperatures. Can stay fresh for up to 3 months.

SELECTING AND STORING FRESH PRODUCE
(continued)

	Selection Tips	Storage Tips
Broccoli	Choose odorless heads with tight, bluish-green florets. Avoid stalks with yellow leaves or florets.	Refrigerate for use within 3–5 days.
Eggplant	Choose eggplants that are heavy for their size and without cracks or discolorations.	Store in the refrigerator crisper drawer. Use within 3–5 days.
Spinach	Choose fresh, green bunches with no yellow leaves.	Loosely wrap in a damp paper towel. Refrigerate in a plastic bag for use within 3–5 days.
Tomato	Choose tomatoes with bright shiny skins and firm flesh.	Store at room temperature away from direct sunlight. Use within 1 week after tomato is ripe. Refrigerate tomatoes only if you can't use them before they spoil.

CANNED FRUITS AND VEGETABLES

When buying canned fruits or vegetables, consider these selection tips:

- *Get the juice.* For canned fruit, look for descriptions on the label like "packed in its own juices," "packed in fruit juice," "unsweetened," or "in syrup." Unsweetened fruits and fruits packed in juice are better choices (containing less added sugar and fewer calories) than fruits packed in syrup.
- *Pinch the salt.* To cut back on sodium, look for descriptions such as "no salt added" and "reduced sodium" on the labels of canned vegetables.

- *Savor the flavor.* For maximum flavor and nutritional value, use canned fruits and vegetables immediately after opening them.

> **Parents Weigh In: Pick Frozen for Peak Nutritional Performance**
>
> I got tired of wasting money and throwing away shriveled-up greens and moldy berries. Now I buy frozen fruits and vegetables. I've heard that they are picked at their peak, which locks in their nutrients.
> —MARIE, MOM OF FOUR CHILDREN

Frozen Fruits and Vegetables

Here are some tips to help you when buying frozen fruits and vegetables:

- *Forgo the fat.* When buying frozen vegetables, control fat and calories by choosing plain vegetables or those made with low-fat sauces.
- *Check the label.* Frozen fruits come in both sweetened and unsweetened varieties, so make sure to check the label and choose unsweetened fruit to cut back on added sugars. Frozen juice bars also make a nutritious snack, but read labels and choose those made with 100 percent fruit juice.

Dried Fruits

Consider these tips when choosing dried fruits:

- *Pick the plain.* Dried fruits provide fiber, vitamins A and C, potassium, and folate. However, they also have more calories per serving than fresh fruit because of their natural, and sometimes added, sugar. Also, some dried fruits are preserved with sulfite, which can trigger allergic reactions in sensitive individuals. Read package labels to make sure your choices are safe for your child or teen and in line with his or her MyPlate daily eating plan.
- *Have a handful.* Dried fruit is a great portable snack. It can also jazz up salad, pancakes, bread recipes, or a bowl of cereal.

The "Dirt" on Fresh Fruits and Vegetables

Many fruits and vegetables come in contact with soil while growing, and they can become contaminated with bacteria that cause foodborne illnesses

WASHING TIPS FOR FRUITS AND VEGGIES

All fresh produce, regardless of where it was grown or purchased, should be thoroughly rinsed. Follow these tips to help ensure that your fruits and vegetables are clean and safe to eat:

- Rinse fresh vegetables and fruits under running water just before eating, cutting, or cooking. Do not use soap or detergent; commercial produce washes are not needed.
- Even if you plan to peel or cut the produce before eating, it's still important to thoroughly rinse it first to prevent microbes from transferring from the outside to the inside of the produce.
- Scrub firm produce, such as melons and cucumbers, with a clean produce brush while you rinse it.
- Dry produce with a clean cloth towel or paper towel to further reduce bacteria that may be present. Wet produce can allow remaining microbes to multiply faster.
- Many precut packaged items, like lettuce or baby carrots, are labeled as prewashed and ready-to-eat. These products can be eaten without further rinsing.

(such as salmonella and E. coli bacteria) if they are not handled properly. However, that risk is not a good reason to avoid giving kids fresh produce. Foodborne illness is easily preventable by properly washing and storing fresh fruits and vegetables (*see* Washing Tips for Fruits and Veggies).

Maximizing the Nutrients in Fruits and Vegetables

For maximum nutritional benefit, most types of fresh fruits and vegetables should be eaten raw and within a few days of purchase. This is because the levels of vitamins and phytonutrients in most produce decrease with cooking and as time passes after harvest. However, tomatoes, carrots, and corn are exceptions to this recommendation. They contain lycopene, and lightly cooking them allows our bodies absorb that phytonutrient more easily.

Kids usually enjoy raw fruit, but getting kids to eat raw vegetables can be a challenge. If your child or teen prefers cooked vegetables, choose one of the following quick-cooking methods, which retain the most flavor, color, and nutrients:

- *Steaming*—Steaming works for most fresh and frozen vegetables, including asparagus, beans, broccoli, carrots, and new potatoes. It's quick, and the high temperature of the steam locks in the nutrients. To steam vegetables on the stovetop, place them in a colander or strainer over a saucepan of boiling water. The vegetables are done when they become crisp-tender. Electric steamers are another option. They are easier to use, and most steaming baskets can do double-duty as serving dishes.
- *Microwaving*—Using a microwave is great for cooking and reheating vegetables because it's fast and you don't need to add extra fat. When you microwave vegetables, use very little water and be sure to cover them with a lid or microwave-safe plastic wrap to keep the steam in the dish.
- *Stir-frying*—Another great cooking method for preserving flavor, color, and nutrients is stir-frying. Cut the vegetables into thin slices so they will heat quickly. Cook them for a few minutes over high heat, ideally in a nonstick skillet or wok; use a little broth or about a teaspoon of oil to keep the vegetables from sticking.

In addition to using quick-cooking methods, here are some other tips to minimize the loss of nutrients from fruits and vegetables:

- *Slice and dice.* Cut thick vegetables that may need to cook longer (such as potatoes or sweet potatoes) into large pieces instead of small ones. Fewer vitamins are lost when fewer surfaces are exposed.
- *Reheat then eat.* Canned vegetables have already been cooked, so just reheat them on the stove or in the microwave instead of cooking them slowly.
- *Save the water!* After cooking or reheating vegetables, make sure you serve them with the cooking water—that's where many of the B vitamins will have migrated. You can also save the nutrient-rich vegetable liquid to serve in soups, stews, and sauces.

- *Add ingredients carefully.* A splash of lemon juice or vinegar will help beets and red cabbage keep their bright color. Never add baking soda to green vegetables! It may keep veggies looking green, but only at the expense of destroying precious vitamins.

Should You Go Organic?

Organic foods are produced without antibiotics, hormones, genetic engineering, radiation, or synthetic pesticides or fertilizers. To label their foods "organic," producers must be certified organic according the regulations of the U.S. Department of Agriculture.

The choice to buy organic or conventional produce is a personal one. To date, there is no conclusive scientific evidence to show that organically produced foods are healthier or safer than conventionally grown foods. Both organic and conventional farming supply nutritionally comparable foods. Organic produce often costs more than conventionally grown foods. However, if you buy it in season or grow your own, it can be equal in price to or less expensive than conventional produce.

> **Kids Weigh In: Organic versus Healthy Eating**
>
> I used to think that eating an organic cookie was healthier for me than eating a non-organic apple.
> —STACIE, AGE 16

To learn more about organic foods, look to the U.S. Department of Agriculture. Its Agricultural Marketing Program Web site *(www.ams.usda.gov)* includes a section on the National Organic Program, which develops, implements, and administers national production, handling, and labeling standards for organic foods. There you can find how the term "organic" can be used on food labels as well as fact sheets that can help you weigh your options.

Learning to Love Fruits and Veggies

Think back to when you were a kid. Was there a vegetable you despised, but now you adore it? Learning to love and eat fruits and veggies is a lifelong process. Research has proven that our eating habits are formed at very early ages. Certain events and practices during our early years may trigger feeding problems that lead to an unhealthy weight. The next topic—Why Are Kids Picky Eaters?—covers issues related to this early stage of development and may be most relevant to parents of children under the age of six. If your child is older, you may want to skim this material and concentrate more on the following section, How to Raise a Fruit and Veggie Lover (page 145).

Why Kids Are Picky Eaters

Being a picky eater can be a natural state for young children. They are born with an instinctive desire for sweet and salty foods, and an instinctive aversion to sour and bitter tastes. These instincts are a trait left over from our "caveman" days. Back then, the reflex to reject sour-bitter foods served as a survival mechanism so that youngsters wouldn't wander off and nibble on poisonous plants and berries—many of which are not sweet. Today, however, this reflex is one of the key reasons so many kids become picky eaters and shun fruits and vegetables. Luckily, kids can eventually overcome this tendency by being repeatedly exposed to foods they initially reject. Just be patient. Offer picky kids some of the sweeter-tasting vegetables, such as carrots, sweet potatoes, and acorn squash, and don't push them to eat more bitter options—such as broccoli, green beans, cauliflower, and dark leafy greens like spinach—if they reject them (but try again another day). Also, make sure fruits are ripe, sweet, and juicy. Hold off on sour or tart fruits like grapefruit or granny smith apples until your child's tastebuds mature.

Kids' natural preference for sweet-salty foods and rejection of bitter-sour foods has a yin-and-yang effect on their eating habits. Researchers call this *neophobia* (fear of trying new foods). Studies have found that neophobia reaches its peak between the ages of two and six years—when rejection of vegetables reaches an all-time high. This phobia explains why children in this stage of development often go on food jags in which they will eat only one or two foods that they like and refuse to eat anything else—like our friend Mario from the beginning of this chapter. Most kids outgrow food jags if parents and other caregivers don't make a big deal about their food preferences (*see* What to Say to Encourage Picky Eaters).

WHAT TO SAY TO ENCOURAGE PICKY EATERS

- **Choose** phrases that help point out the sensory qualities of food, like "This kiwi fruit is sweet like a strawberry" or "These radishes are very crunchy!" They encourage your child to try new foods.
- **Avoid** phrases that teach your child to eat for approval and love, like "Eat that for me" or "If you do not eat one more bite, I will be mad." This can lead your child to have unhealthy behaviors, attitudes, and beliefs about food and about themselves.
- **Choose** phrases that help your child recognize when he or she is full, like "Is your stomach telling you that you're full?" "Is your stomach still making its hungry growling noise?" "Has your tummy had enough?" These statements can help prevent overeating.
- **Avoid** phrases that encourage kids to ignore signs of fullness, like "You're such a big girl; you finished all your peas," "Look at your sister. She ate all of her bananas," or "You have to take one more bite before you leave the table."
- **Choose** phrases that make your child feel like he or she is making the choices, like "Do you like that?" "Which one is your favorite?" or "Everyone likes different foods, don't they?" These statements shift the focus toward the taste of food rather than who was right.
- **Avoid** phrases that imply a child was wrong to refuse a food, like "See, that didn't taste so bad, did it?" These statements can lead to unhealthy attitudes about food or self.
- **Choose** phrases that comfort or reward your child with attention and kind words, like "I am sorry you are sad. Come here and let me give you a big hug." Show love by spending time and having fun together.
- **Avoid** phrases that make some foods seem like a comfort, like "Stop crying and I will give you a cookie." Getting a food treat when upset teaches your child to eat to feel better. This can cause overeating.

(continued)

WHAT TO SAY TO ENCOURAGE PICKY EATERS
(continued)

- **Avoid** phrases that make foods seem like a reward or like they are better than other foods, such as "No dessert until you eat your vegetables." A better way to encourage your child to keep trying vegetables might be, "We can try these vegetables again another time. Next time would you like to them raw instead of cooked?"

Adapted from MyPlate: Phrases that Help and Hinder poster.
www.choosemyplate.gov/preschoolers/HealthyHabits/phrasesthathelp.pdf.

If you're concerned that your child's or teen's picky eating has lasted too long or is very restrictive, seek help from an RD. However, parents of picky preschoolers may also take some comfort in knowing that several studies show that infants and young children know how much they need to eat. In the 1930s, researcher Clara Davis presented infants and young children with a variety of nutritious foods and allowed them to self-select what they ate, in the absence of their parents, and the kids remained healthy and grew normally. Several other studies have repeated her experiment with the same results. If a child eats a large breakfast, he or she is hard-wired to eat less at dinner or lunch. Unfortunately, many kids lose this calorie-balancing instinct somewhere along the way—typically around age five. Rather than eat because they are hungry and stop because they are full, kids learn to eat because of outside influences such as super-size portions and a steady stream of snack food commercials on television. And, unlike the children in Ms. Davis's research lab, kids in the real world are offered more than nutritious choices. They're surrounded by candy, soft drinks, fast food, and other temptations. The bottom line: it is our job as parents to help our kids get back in touch with their appetites, provide them with healthy food options, especially fruits and vegetables, and let them choose which ones and how much to eat.

How to Raise a Fruit and Veggie Lover

Even though eating habits are formed when we are younger, it's never too late to learn how to eat healthy for a healthy weight. Kids of all ages (even adults) can learn to change and improve their eating habits. And, with time and loving patience, kids can acquire a taste for not-so-favorite foods. Here are some strategies for getting kids to eat healthier and enjoy more fruits and veggies:

- *Parents—eat your veggies!* When you are a good role model, you'll produce better results in your kids. Make sure you eat fruits and veggies *and* make sure your child or teen sees you eating and enjoying them.
- *Start early.* Moms, eat a wide variety of fruits and veggies when you're pregnant and nursing. Studies have found that fetuses and breastfed infants experience the flavors of the maternal diet before their first exposure to these flavors in solid foods. This early exposure may lead to an earlier acceptance of these foods.
- *Try it, you'll like it.* Kids are reluctant to try new foods, but the more often a food is presented (even if it's not eaten), the more positive a kid's attitude will be toward the food. It can take up to 10 offerings before some kids will even put a new food in their mouth! So don't give up too early. Be patient and keep offering the food. You can also try serving it different ways. For example, offer broccoli with a dip, broccoli steamed with a drizzle of cheese sauce, broccoli diced and tossed in pasta sauce, and broccoli soup.
- *Taste first, swallowing is optional.* When encouraging kids to taste new foods, establish the "taste-but-don't-have-to-swallow" policy. Let kids know that there is no need to make yucky faces or cause a scene if they don't like the taste of a certain fruit or vegetable. Give

them a small portion to taste; if they don't care for the food, they
can politely use a paper napkin to remove it from their mouth.

- *Conduct "either/or" negotiations.* Encourage kids to choose the fruits
  and vegetables they eat, but don't overwhelm them with endless
  fruit and vegetable options. Kids will feel more empowered if you
  give them forced-choice options such as: Would you like a sweet
  potato or carrots for dinner? How does watermelon sound for a
  snack or would you prefer sliced peaches?

- *Offer new foods first.* Introduce kids to a new fruit or vegetable by
  serving it at the beginning of the meal when they're more likely to
  be hungry. You can also put a plate of bell pepper strips, baby carrots, and peapods on the counter when you're preparing lunch or
  dinner and let kids nibble. This helps take the edge off their appetite in a healthy way, and it will help them reach their veggie
  quota.

- *Serve veggies and fruit family-style.* Dish up kids' plates with recommended servings from each of the MyPlate food groups (*see* Chapter 3), but keep a bowl of vegetables and fruits on the table for
  passing. If kids want seconds, they can have more fruits and vegetables. It's a great way to help kids get in touch with their appetite
  and reach a healthy weight.

- *Give your kids a say when shopping.* Bring kids with you to the grocery store or a farmer's market and let them pick which fruits and
  vegetables they want to try. Older kids can go on a scavenger hunt.
  Give them a list of fresh produce and have them search for the
  items.

- *Make fruits and veggies convenient.* Fruits such as bananas, apples,
  oranges, and grapes are the healthiest "fast foods"—they come
  packed in their very own containers! Keep them in a bowl on the
  counter for a quick snack. Also, keep a stash of washed, peeled,
  and sliced fruits and veggies at eye-level in refrigerator. Time savers
  like prepackaged salads and bags of baby carrots and apple wedges
  are worth the extra money if kids eat them instead of chips or
  cookies.

- *Avoid rewards and bribes.* Kids are too smart to fall for the "if you eat your spinach, you can have dessert" trick. Studies show that this approach to offering fruits and vegetables—or really any food—sets the healthier option up for failure.
- *Stand firm.* If kids won't eat their kiwi or peas, don't fight with them. Tell them that's fine, but they will not be able to eat anything until the next meal. Many kids crave the extra attention they get from not eating. Refusing to battle with them often motivates kids to eat.
- *Tell favorite veggie tales.* Let kids know what your favorite fruit or vegetable is and why. Share with them the first time you ate it and who was with you. Give them an opportunity to share their favorites, too.
- *Grow a vegetable garden.* Studies find that kids who grow their own fruits and vegetables are more likely to eat them. Try planting seeds in your backyard or indoors in pots or greenhouses. For tips, visit the Centers for Disease Control and Prevention's Web page "Spring Seedlings: Tips for Growing Your Own Vegetables" *(www.cdc.gov/Features/GrowingVegetables).*
- *Prepare for limited options.* Family road trips, amusement parks, movie theaters—fruits and veggies can be hard to find when kids are the go. Fill a cooler or backpack with grapes, pears, raisins, and baby carrots to make sure they'll get to pick some produce.

Should Kids "Veg" Out?

If your child wants to become a vegetarian, there's no need to panic. According to the Academy of Nutrition and Dietetics, a well-planned vegetarian diet is appropriate for all people at all stages of life, and this includes growing children and teens. However, the key phrase here is *well-planned.* Candy bars and soft drinks qualify as vegetarian fare, but they are, of course, not health foods. A registered dietitian can help you and your son or daughter design a vegetarian eating plan that provides needed nutrients and is high in fiber, low in solid fat and cholesterol, and conducive to promoting a healthy weight (*see* I'm a Vegetarian! on page 148).

I'M A VEGETARIAN!

So your child or teen wants to give the vegetarian lifestyle a try? It's important to ask what type of vegetarian. While all vegetarians exclude meat, some eat certain animal products, such as milk and eggs, and some do not:

- *Lacto-ovo vegetarians* eat dairy and egg products (this is the most nutritious vegetarian choice for growing teens).
- *Lacto-vegetarians* eat dairy products but do not eat eggs.
- *Ovo-vegetarians* eat eggs but do not eat dairy products.
- *Vegans* eat food from plant sources only; they do not eat eggs, dairy products, or honey.

Vegetarians need to eat a well-planned diet to ensure they get enough of the following key nutrients: protein, vitamin B-12, vitamin D, calcium, iron, and zinc. Young vegetarians should always work with a registered dietitian.

The Garden of Eatin'—Getting Kids to Eat the Recommended Daily Amount of Fruits and Vegetables

Getting kids to eat fruits and vegetables is both a science and art. So far, you've mostly learned about the science. Now let's talk about the art. There are many ways to easily and creatively incorporate fruits and veggies into every meal and snack. You'll also find several quick and tasty fruit and vegetable recipes in Chapter 11.

Breakfast

Fruit fits easily into breakfast, but vegetables can be a challenge. Here are some tips to help you wake up your kid's fruit and vegetable appetite:

- *Stir things up.* For a quick breakfast, add raisins or chopped dates to instant oatmeal or stir blueberries, strawberries, or sliced banana into whole grain cereal with fat-free milk.

- *Get scrambling!* Add fresh or frozen chopped spinach, mushrooms, and diced tomatoes to scrambled eggs or omelets. Really, any veggies will work!
- *Make a breakfast sandwich.* Top a whole wheat English muffin with either reduced-fat peanut butter and banana slices or a poached egg, a slice of Canadian bacon, and a pineapple ring.
- *Batter up.* Add grated carrots or zucchini to pancake, quick bread, or muffin batter.
- *Drink your produce.* Whir carrots and fresh orange juice in a blender for a refreshing breakfast beverage.
- *Say "Olé!"* Make a breakfast burrito by wrapping low-fat cheddar cheese, scrambled eggs, and diced bell peppers in a whole wheat tortilla. You can also make a vegetable and cheese quesadilla in a nonstick pan with a scant amount of canola oil.
- *Pick a fruit pizza.* Spread reduced-fat dinner rolls in a pizza pan and bake. Top the pizza with orange sections or slices of kiwi, apples, or strawberries and drizzle fat-free vanilla yogurt over the top.
- *Make a quick white or sweet potato hash.* Grate the potatoes—they cook faster that way. Place the potatoes in a glass bowl and microwave about three minutes or until hot; drain any juice. Heat a skillet or frying pan on the stove and then stir-fry the potatoes with a teaspoon of olive oil until crispy.

Lunch

Kids eat lunch everywhere—at home, daycare, and school. Some buy lunch; others brown-bag it. Here are some tips to help you make sure lunch includes fruits and vegetables:

- *Quick and easy.* Capitalize on healthy convenience foods. Look for prepackaged baby carrots and dip, pineapple slices, mini-boxes of raisins or dried fruit, and single-serve cans of fruit like diced peaches and pears packed in juice. (To save money, you can also make your own grab-and-go, single-serving packages.)
- *Shake it up, baby!* Fill a plastic container with lettuce, diced bell peppers, dried cranberries, and chickpeas—or any diced fruit or

veggie—and drizzle a small amount of fat-free ranch dressing on top. Tell your child to shake it up and enjoy. For a more complete lunch, add diced chicken breast or ham and fat-free whole grain croutons.

- *Give them the right stuff.* Stuff a whole grain pita pocket with leftover roasted veggies. Eggplant, bell peppers, zucchini, and onions are easy to grill and hold up well in a lunchbox or bag. Or make tuna or chicken salad with finely diced veggies like green onion, celery, or jicama and blend of fat-free or low-fat plain yogurt and fat-free mayo (for a fruity twist, add grapes or pineapple tidbits, too).

- *Slurp their veggies.* For lunch at school, fill a thermos with hot veg-etable soup, or pack a frozen vegetable juice box—it will thaw by lunch and be ready for sipping.

- *Send fruity love notes.* Make fresh fruit more appealing. Draw a fun-ny face or write a joke or friendly reminder (soccer @ 2 PM!) on a banana or orange peel for kids to see.

- *Peanut butter and no jelly!* Instead of jelly, add sweetness to a peanut butter sandwich with pear or apple slices, raisins, or sliced grapes.

Snacks

Snack attacks are a reality for growing kids (*see* Chapter 3). Here are some tips to make sure they're nibbling on fruits and veggies:

- *Build incredible edibles.* Place an assortment of precut veggies and fruits in a stay-fresh container. Using reduced-fat peanut butter and their imagination, let kids build a variety of creations such as smiley faces, butterflies, kites—whatever looks and sounds tasty.

- *Take a hike.* Kids love trail mix. Combine whole grain cereal, dried cranberries, chopped almonds, and sunflower seeds. Be sure to make a big batch and divide it into single-size portions.

- *Dip it!* Dip sliced jicama strips, carrots, celery sticks, or other crunchy veggies into salsa or hummus (chickpea spread). Hummus also tastes terrific on whole grain pita bread.

- *Scoop up a yogurt or pudding parfait.* Skip the ice cream. Instead, kids can layer fat-free yogurt and fresh berries into a sundae dish.

Sugar-free pudding made with fat-free milk also makes a tasty base for this sort of fruit parfait.

- *Hot potato!* Zap a baked potato in the microwave and top it with cooked fresh or frozen broccoli florets and shredded low-fat cheddar cheese.
- *Nibble on pizza bites.* Top mini whole grain bagels with tomato sauce, shredded low-fat mozzarella cheese, and chopped veggies such as bell peppers, mushrooms, and onions. Pop the pizzas into a toaster oven for about 10 minutes—chow!

Dinner

What's for dinner? Whether it's at home or at a restaurant, here are some tips to make sure fruits and veggies are part of the menu:

- *Pizza pizazz.* Skip the meat and order pizza with extra veggies like bell peppers, mushrooms, tomatoes, and onions. For a tropical twist try a Hawaiian pizza with pineapple and lean ham.
- *Thrill with the grill.* Cut potatoes, carrots, corn on the cob, zucchini and eggplant into smaller chunks. Wrap them in foil and grill for about 10 to 15 minutes. Serve them with a splash of olive oil and seasoning (*see* Veggie Seasonings on page 152).
- *Make "mock" spaghetti.* Use spaghetti squash instead of pasta. Simply bake or microwave the spaghetti squash in its shell until it is tender. Run a fork through the squash to tear it to shreds—it will look just like spaghetti. Add your favorite tomato sauce and toss in other veggies, like onions and sweet bell pepper. For a southwestern flavor, use salsa and toss in black beans, corn kernels and red, yellow, and green bell peppers.
- *Serve up salsa.* Liven up a lean cut of meat, like flank steak or pork tenderloin, with a salsa made from diced fruits and vegetables. For a Mediterranean flair, combine cucumber, grape tomatoes, red onion, fresh dill, red wine vinegar, and a splash of olive oil. Or go tropical by tossing green bell pepper, pineapple, sweet onion, and mango with fresh lime juice. In a hurry? Pick up a jar of salsa from the supermarket.

VEGGIE SEASONINGS

Vegetable	Delicious Seasoning Options
Asparagus	Garlic, fresh lemon juice, onion, vinegar
Beans	Caraway, cloves, cumin, mint, savory, tarragon, thyme
Beets	Anise, caraway, fennel, ginger, savory
Carrots	Anise, cinnamon, cloves, mint, sage, tarragon
Corn	Allspice, chili powder, dill
Cucumbers	Chives, dill, garlic, vinegar
Green beans	Dill, fresh lemon juice, marjoram, nutmeg
Greens	Garlic, fresh lemon juice, onion, vinegar
Peas	Allspice, mint, fresh mushroom, onion, parsley, sage, savory
Potatoes	Chives, dill, onion, saffron, sage
Tomatoes	Allspice, basil, garlic, marjoram, onion, oregano, sage, savory, tarragon, thyme
Winter squash (butternut, acorn, etc.)	Allspice, cinnamon, cloves, fennel, ginger, mace, nutmeg, onion, savory

Healthy Eating, Healthy Weight—You're in Control

■ *Mario's parents met with the RD, Donna, who helped them work through some of their son's picky eating issues and set family-focused goals to break the pattern of pandering to Mario's food demands. They filled out a family contract to remind them not to give in to Mario and stick with their goals:*

We, the Valentine family, will work toward the following goal(s) over the next one or two weeks: (1) Offer Mario a fruit or vegetable at every meal and snack. (2) Let Mario decide how much he wants to eat. (3) Serve as good role models by eating a fruit or vegetable at every meal and snack. When we have successfully made these a habit, we will reward ourselves with making a Saturday trip to the country to go apple picking. Signed: Mario (Sr.), Marie, and Mario Valentine.

Instead of offering food bribes, Mario's parents now offer him a taste of a colorful fruit or vegetable at the beginning of each meal, when he is most likely to be hungry, and Mario gets to decide how much he wants to eat. If he likes the fruit or vegetable, he can ask for more. Mario's parents make it a point to eat and talk about fruits and vegetables with Mario. They also take Mario to the supermarket so he can see fresh produce—he loves when the sprinklers come on to mist the vegetables and splash him if he gets too close! Mom went online to the Fruit and Veggie Color Champions Web site (http://www.foodchamps.org) *and printed fruit and vegetable rainbow activity sheets for Mario to color. Mario is now meeting his daily MyPlate target of one cup of fruits and one cup of vegetables. Since he's been eating more fruits and veggies, he's no longer filling up on higher calorie foods like cookies and French fries. His healthy eating is helping him reach a healthy weight.* ■

Getting kids to eat fruits and vegetables is a challenge most parents face. But the research is clear: kids who eat the most fruits and vegetables are less likely to be overweight. To help your child or teen to be a healthy weight, it is important to follow *Healthy Eating, Healthy Weight Strategy #5: Fill up on fruits and veggies! Eat plenty of servings of fruits and vegetables every day.*

In this chapter, you have explored a variety of options to help kids learn to enjoy eating a colorful plate full of fruits and vegetables. Now it's time to set some goals as a family and write a family goal contract (*see* the sample form at the end of Chapter 2). Here are a few examples of goals to get you started:

- Eat (or at least try) a fruit or vegetable at every meal and snack.
- Go to a weekend farmer's market with your family.
- Try one new fruit and one new vegetable this week.
- Have every family member keep a fruit and vegetable calendar.
- Place a bowl of fruit on the kitchen counter and a bag of cut of veggies in the refrigerator for easy snacking.

Keep tabs of your family's progress by completing a tracking card similar to the one at the end of Chapter 2. After your family accomplishes the first goals, continue to come up with creative and fun ways to include more fruits and vegetables in meals and snack until everyone is meeting the targets in their MyPlate daily food plan. Your family will reap the benefits!

8

Healthy Eating, Healthy Weight Strategy #6: Slow Down the Fast Food!

■ *Eleven-year-old twins Lauren and Lindsey Anderson play competitive soccer year-round. Busy with practice, games, and weekend tournaments, the Andersons eat fast food at least four times a week, sometimes even for breakfast. Lauren is not too crazy about fast food, but Lindsey loves it. She usually orders a double cheeseburger, large fries, and an extra-large milkshake. Up until this year, the twins were always on the same soccer team. However, this season Lauren made the A team while Lindsey made the B team. A disappointed Lindsey said she wanted to quit. The twins' parents had noticed that Lindsey had gained a lot of weight in the past six months and become much slower on the soccer field. Their mom therefore decided to set up an appointment for Lindsey with a registered dietitian (RD). After thoroughly assessing Lindsey's eating and physical activity habits, the RD recommended that the family follow* Healthy Eating, Healthy Weight Strategy #6: Slow down the fast food! Eat fast food less than once a week. ■

Your meeting ran late, the dry cleaner closes at 6 PM, and the kids have back-to-back Little League games. Who has time to sit down and eat dinner? Compared to years past, Americans spend 45 percent less time preparing food at home or eating food at the family table. Many busy families have come to rely on fast food, especially because value meal deals are quick and budget-friendly. However, studies show that eating too much fast food can speed up unhealthy weight gain for both kids and adults. For example, soccer-playing Lindsey requires about 1,600 calories a day to be a healthy weight (*see* Chapter 3), but her usual fast-food meal provides about 1,800 calories all on its own! If your family, like the Andersons, is spending more time at the drive-through window than around the dinner table, this chapter will help you slow down the fast food and learn how your family can eat healthy even when they're in a hurry.

Fast Food: The Weight Debate

All types of food—even fast food—can fit into a healthy eating plan. In fact, many fast-food chains now offer healthier options such as low-fat milk and apple slices, and, as we'll discuss in this chapter, kids can enjoy a fast-food hamburger and French fries every once in awhile. However, compared to meals at home, fast-food meal are usually short on the vegetables, fruits, low-fat or fat-free dairy foods, and whole grains that provide nutrients of particular importance for growing children and teens, such as calcium, vitamin D, vitamin A, vitamin C, fiber, and phytonutrients (compounds that may help fight or prevent certain diseases like cancer).

Kids Weigh In: Fast Food Equals Fattening Food!

I watched a movie in health class about all the calories and fat in fast food. I'm going to think about that the next time I go out to eat with friends.

—KEVIN, AGE 14

Furthermore, as you can see by taking the Your Order Please! Quiz, fast-food meals tend to be high in calories, sodium (salt), and fat (especially the "bad" types, saturated and *trans* fats). This is a Healthy Weight concern because in recent years fast food has changed from an occasional treat to an everyday meal for many Americans. On any given day, about one-third of kids between the ages of 4 and 19 eat fast food, and the typical tween or teen eats at fast-food chains twice a week. These fast-food habits have consequences for our kids' weight and health. Studies have found that kids who eat fast food are at an increased risk of becoming overweight and obese—particularly if they eat one or more fast-food meals a week.

YOUR ORDER PLEASE! QUIZ

Take a look at these pairs of fast-food options that seem to be on the lighter side. From each pair, try to pick the menu item with the *least* amount of calories, fat, and sodium.

Quiz

Fast-Food Option A	Fast-Food Option B
1 1 regular-size hamburger	1 small taco
2 Large taco salad with shell	2 bean burritos
3 Grilled chicken breast sandwich	6-inch turkey sub
4 1 cup chili con carne	1 cup broccoli-cheddar soup
5 6 chicken nuggets	Fish sandwich with tartar sauce
6 1 slice thin-and-crispy cheese pizza	1 slice thick-crust cheese pizza

Answer Key: 1A (1 regular-size hamburger = 275 calories, 12 grams [g] fat, 385 milligrams [mg] sodium; 1 small taco = 370 calories, 21 g fat, 800 mg sodium). **2B** (large taco salad with shell = 905 calories, 49 g fat, 1,935 mg sodium; 2 bean burritos = 447 calories, 14 g fat, 985 mg sodium). **3B** (grilled chicken breast sandwich = 419 calories, 10 g fat, 1, 235 mg sodium; 6-inch turkey sub = 280 calories, 3.5 g fat, 920 mg sodium). **4A** (1 cup chili con carne = 255 calories, 8 g fat, 1,010 mg sodium; 1 cup broccoli-cheddar soup = 290 calories, 16 g fat, 1,540 mg sodium). **5A** (6 chicken nuggets = 285 calories, 18 g fat, 550 mg sodium; fish sandwich with tartar sauce = 430 calories, 23 g fat, 615 mg sodium). **6A** (1 slice thin-and-crispy cheese pizza = 210 calories, 10 g fat, 540 mg sodium; 1 slice thick-crust pizza = 280 calories, 12.5 g fat, 625 mg sodium).

How to Interpret Your Score

Give yourself one point for each correct answer. How did you score?
0–3: Uh, oh! Time to start paying attention to fast-food calorie and nutrition information.
4–5: Not bad! Keep paying attention to fast-food calorie and nutrition information.
6: Great! Knowing fast-food calorie and nutrition information can help your child or teen reach and maintain a healthy weight.

Family Life in the Fast-Food Lane

To achieve and maintain a healthy weight, kids should ideally eat fast food, including fast food breakfasts, no more than three times a month (*see* Fast-Food Breakfast: An Eye-Opening Meal). However, we all know that fast food is a reality for many busy families. If your family eats fast food, the key is to become informed customers. To make healthier choices, kids need to know how many calories and how much fat and sodium is in that slice of cheesy pizza or triple bacon burger *before* they order (*see* Anatomy of a Fast-Food Burger).

FAST-FOOD BREAKFAST: AN EYE-OPENING EXPERIENCE

Many kids start their day eating fast food. The good news: they're eating breakfast, which is a very important meal (*see* Chapter 9). The bad news: fast-food breakfast options are high in calories, fat, and sodium. Here are a few suggestions for lightening up your kid's fast-food breakfast picks.

Instead of:	Order:
Egg sandwich on a croissant or biscuit	Egg sandwich on an English muffin
Egg sandwich with sausage or bacon	Egg sandwich with Canadian bacon
Pancakes with butter and syrup	Pancakes with jam
Breakfast burrito with cheese and sausage	Breakfast burrito with eggs, bell peppers, and salsa
French toast sticks and syrup	English muffin with jam
Cinnamon bun	Yogurt fruit parfait
Soft drink	Orange juice
Whole or reduced-fat (2%) milk	Low-fat (1%) or fat-free (skim) milk

ANATOMY OF A FAST-FOOD BURGER

Kids may dream about a triple bacon cheese burger with all of the fixings, but adding certain ingredients to a basic fast-food burger can quickly load the meal with calories, fat, and salt.

Burger Ingredient	Calories	Fat	Sodium
Bun	120	1 gram	240 mg
Single patty	220	15 grams	170 mg
Double patty	440	30 grams	340 mg
Triple patty	660	45 grams	510 mg
Cheese (1 slice)	70	5 grams	320 mg
Ketchup (1 tablespoon)	15	0 grams	165 mg
Mustard (1 tablespoon)	10	0 grams	170 mg
Mayonnaise (1 tablespoon)	55	5 grams	105 mg

Data are from Fast Food Facts Web site. *www.fastfoodfacts.info.*

Fast Food—Get the Facts

Nowadays, major fast-food restaurants provide nutrition information about menu items on their corporate Web sites and they are required by law to list the calorie content of standard menu items on their menus and menu boards, even at the drive-through. Several Web sites also allow you to quickly compare fast-food menu options from a variety of local and national chains: try Healthy Dining Finder *(www.healthydiningfinder.com),* Fast Food Nutrition Facts *(www.fastfoodnutrition.org),* Diet Facts *(www .dietfacts.com),* or Fast Food Facts *(www.fastfoodfacts.info).* Also, you and your tweens and teens can download fast-food nutrition apps to your cellphones.

Fast-Food Tips to Help Kids Eat on the Go

Burgers, pizza, or tacos—no matter what types of fast food kids prefer, healthy weight choices are available. In addition to checking the nutrition facts for specific fast foods, keep the following ordering tips in mind when you and your kids are scanning the menu board:

- *Look for "light" menu items.* Most chains offer at least a few lower calorie choices and will often feature them on the menu board under catchy names such as "fit" or "fresco." Note: Some chains feature organic meats, but these are not necessarily lower in calories.

- *Come to "terms" with cooking options.* Pass up foods that are deep-fried, especially if they are breaded and coated (such as fried chicken or fried fish filets). For fewer calories, choose fast foods that are broiled, grilled, baked, or stir-fried.

- *Downsize portions.* Choose the regular-size portion rather than the double, triple, or super-deluxe option. The larger the portion, the more calories, fat, and sodium (*see* Chapter 6). Also, regardless of your child's age, go ahead and order a kiddie meal. They come in smaller portions and include healthier sides (*see* Healthy Kiddie Meals Make Parents Happy on page 162).

- *Be slather savvy.* Order burgers and sandwiches without the mayonnaise or special sauce. Depending on the portion, these sauces can add from 10 to 400 extra calories. If your child wants the flavor of the condiment, order it on the side and let him or her spread on a tiny amount. Better yet, use lower calorie sauces such as mustard or ketchup.

- *Pile on healthy extras.* Load fast food with fresh veggies whenever possible. Order pizza with peppers, mushrooms, and tomatoes. Stuff some lettuce, onions, dill pickle, and tomato slices into burgers, sandwiches, and wraps.

- *Find some fiber.* Many fast-food restaurants offer whole grain buns, tortillas, and pizza crust; whole wheat noodles; and brown rice. Ask for these options, even if they aren't on the menu. Also, baked potatoes provide fiber, especially in the skin. Any dish with beans will provide fiber, too.

- *Be salad smart.* When salads are drenched in salad dressing, they can have more calories than French fries. Ask for fat-free salad dressing. Also, keep in mind that tuna and chicken salads made with regular mayonnaise are high in fat and calories.

- *Slurp smart.* Fast-food restaurants offer a variety of soups and chilies. The lowest calorie soups are broth-based and made with vegetables and beans. Creamy soups are usually loaded with calories because they are made with whole milk, cheese, and butter. A small bowl of chili is usually a lower calorie choice than a burger or hot dog.
- *Moo-ve away from soft drinks.* Encourage kids to order fat-free or low-fat milk or just drink water. Some chains offer 100 percent fruit juice, too. As a last resort, diet soft-drinks are better than regular, sugar-sweetened soft drinks, but neither type provides any nutrients (*see* Chapter 5).
- *Shake off sodium.* Because of the way they are processed, fast foods are notoriously high in sodium (salt). You can ask that fries and burgers be prepared without added salt, but it's almost impossible to lower the sodium level of fast food to stay within the daily limits recommended in the Dietary Guidelines for Americans (*see* Chapter 3). When your child does eat fast food, make sure the rest of his or her meals that day are lower in sodium.
- *Let them play.* Choose fast-food restaurants that offer a play space where kids can get some physical activity to help burn off any excess calories (*see* Chapter 5).
- *Fill in nutritional gaps.* If you know you'll be stopping to eat fast food while on the road, bring along apples, oranges, or bananas. Fresh fruit is the original fast food—it comes conveniently packed in its own container!

Fast-Food Survival Strategies

Most fast-food chains fall into one of six major categories—burgers, fried chicken, deli, pizza/Italian, Mexican, or Asian—and because each category has its own potential high-calorie pitfalls and lower calorie options, we'll explore them one at a time. For each type of fast-food chain, check out the kid-friendly, quick-pick menu recommendations in the Weighing Your Options charts. Each quick-pick meal provides foods from at least three

HEALTHY KIDDIE MEALS MAKE PARENTS HAPPY

Kiddie meals are usually smaller portions, but they still tend to include foods loaded with fat, sugar, and calories. Here some tips for turning these meals into healthier fare:

- Ask for healthy substitutions (fruit or carrot sticks instead of fries or chips; low-fat or fat-free milk instead of pop; salsa or mustard instead of mayonnaise).
- Talk with your child before ordering a meal so you can agree on the substitutions.
- Make your own home version of a "kiddie" meal. You can even add a sticker or fun note.

Here are a few sample kiddie menus with healthier choices:

- Small turkey sub, baked chips, and water or 100 percent juice
- Chicken nuggets, fruit cup, and low-fat milk
- Small plain hamburger (skip the cheese), yogurt parfait, and water

food groups and is less than 500 calories, making these meals good choices for hungry kids who want to be a healthy weight.

Fast-Food Burger Chains

Nowadays, fast-food burger chains feature more than hamburgers. You'll find everything from chicken to chili to salads on the menu (*see* Weighing Your Options at Burger Chains). Stick with the smallest size burger, or a grilled chicken or grilled fish sandwich, and top it with veggies. Ask for a whole grain bun whenever that is an option. Instead of fries, order a small salad with fat-free dressing, a fresh fruit cup, baby carrots, or a plain baked potato. Skip dessert unless soft-serve ice cream is on the menu—it's lower in fat than regular ice cream and provides some bone-building calcium.

WEIGHING YOUR OPTIONS AT BURGER CHAINS

Instead of:	Order:
Double- and triple-patty hamburgers	Regular, single patty, or junior burger
Fried chicken sandwich	Grilled chicken sandwich with no mayonnaise
Fried chicken nuggets or tenders	Grilled chicken strips
Fried fish sandwich	Grilled fish sandwich without tartar sauce
Extras such as cheese, mayonnaise, special sauce, nuts, or bacon	Extras such as lettuce, tomato, dill pickles, and onion
Salad with toppings such as bacon, cheese, nuts, or regular dressing	Salad with grilled chicken and fat-free or low-fat dressing
French fries	Baked potato (plain)
Milkshakes	Soft-serve ice cream or frozen yogurt

Quick-Pick Menus for Kids*

Hamburger (regular size) with bun, topped with lettuce, tomato, onion, and mustard; French fries (small—split them!); and a carton of low-fat (1%) milk

or

Cheeseburger (regular size) with bun, topped with ketchup and mustard; a side salad with fat-free dressing; a soft-serve ice cream cone (small); and water or a diet soft drink

*Each Quick-Pick menu has less than 500 calories and contains at least three food groups.

FAST-FOOD FRIED CHICKEN CHAINS

Price-wise, it's hard to beat the family chicken meal-deal, but fried chicken is one of the most high-calorie and fattening fast-food options out there! Look for chains that offer grilled chicken. Taking the skin off trims almost

WEIGHING YOUR OPTIONS AT FRIED CHICKEN CHAINS

Instead of:	Order:
Fried chicken	Fried chicken with skin removed or grilled chicken
Potpies or bowls	BBQ chicken sandwich or wrap
Fried chicken strips, popcorn chicken, or wings	Grilled chicken strips
Fried chicken sandwich	Roasted chicken sandwich without mayo
Biscuit or corn bread	Corn on the cob or green beans
Extra gravy or sauces	Fat-free dressing; or use a small amount of BBQ dipping sauce
Coleslaw	Garden salad with fat-free or low-fat dressing or green bean salad
Potato salad or macaroni salad	Mashed potatoes (without gravy)
Macaroni and cheese	Baked beans

Quick-Pick Menu for Kids*

Fried chicken breast or thigh (without skin and breading), mashed potatoes (small serving, hold the gravy), corn on the cob, and a carton of low-fat milk

or

Grilled chicken sandwich on a whole grain bun with lettuce, tomato, and honey-dijon mustard; three bean salad; an apple from home; and water or a diet soft drink

*Each Quick-Pick menu has less than 500 calories and contains at least three food groups.

half the calories. Make sure you choose some of the lighter side dishes, such as corn on the cob, green beans, bean salad, and mashed potatoes without gravy. Baked beans are a high-protein and high-fiber side that could do double-duty as an entrée. Take a pass on desserts such as pie or brownies; most contain too many calories from added fat and sugar. For more advice about ordering, *see* Weighing Your Options at Fried Chicken Chains.

FAST-FOOD DELI CHAINS

Delis and sandwich shops are potentially the healthiest fast-food restaurants—*if* you avoid the larger-than-life portions (*see* Weighing Your Options at Fast-Food Delis). The best way to avoid a deli disaster is to split your order. Many delis feature a combination meal with half a sandwich and a small soup or salad; this option can save money and calories. Load sandwiches with extra veggies and fat-free mustard. Skip the bread bowl if you order soup or a salad—it contains up to 600 calories! On the side, order a bag of baked chips, low-fat yogurt, or fresh fruit.

WEIGHING YOUR OPTIONS AT FAST-FOOD DELIS

Instead of:	Order:
12-inch sub	6-inch sub
High-fat meats, such as meatballs, steak, salami, bacon, tuna salad, and chicken salad	Lean meats, such as roast beef, turkey breast, grilled chicken breast, or lean ham; or veggies
Cheese	Lower fat cheese
Mayonnaise, high-fat special sauces	Low-fat dressing, vinegar, mustard and lots of veggies (lettuce, onion, tomato, cucumber, bell peppers, mushrooms, and pickles)

(continued)

WEIGHING YOUR OPTIONS
AT FAST-FOOD DELIS *(continued)*

Instead of:	Order:
Creamy soups, such as potato, broccoli, or cream of tomato	Broth-based soups, such as chicken noodle or vegetable
Salad with toppings such as bacon, cheese, nuts, and regular dressing	Salad with grilled chicken or shrimp and fat-free or low-fat dressing
Potato chips	Baked chips or pretzels
Cookie or cake	Fresh fruit cup or an apple

Quick-Pick Menu for Kids*

Turkey sub (6-inch) with veggies and vinegar; baked chips (small bag); a fruit cup; and bottled water

or

Garden fresh salad (small or half order) with grilled shrimp and fat-free dressing, a cup vegetable soup, a whole grain roll (small); and water or a diet soft drink

*Each Quick-Pick menu has less than 500 calories and contains at least three food groups.

FAST-FOOD PIZZA AND ITALIAN FOOD CHAINS

Hands down, the most popular fast food for kids is pizza. For the healthiest pizza, order a thin crust (whole grain, if available), scale back the cheese and meat, and pile on the veggies. Salad is a light and healthy side when served with just a splash of oil and vinegar dressing. When ordering pasta, stick with marinara (tomato) sauce and see whether you can substitute whole wheat noodles to add some hunger-filling fiber. For more ordering tips, *see* Weighing Your Options at Pizza/Italian Food Chains.

WEIGHING YOUR OPTIONS AT PIZZA/ITALIAN FOOD CHAINS

Instead of:	Order:
Thick-crust or stuffed-crust pizza with sausage	Thin-crust pizza with half the cheese and extra veggies
Garlic bread	Bread sticks
Antipasto with fatty meats like salami	Antipasto with vegetables
Pasta with cream- or butter-based sauces	Pasta with marinara sauce and veggies
Italian sausage and meatball sandwich	Italian beef sandwich
Pasta noodles (spaghetti, ziti, penne) made with white flour	Whole wheat pasta noodles

Quick-Pick Menu for Kids*

2 slices veggie pizza (thin crust), a side salad with fat-free dressing, and water or a diet soft drink

or

Italian beef sandwich (half order) with peppers, a cup of minestrone soup, and a carton of low-fat milk

*Each Quick-Pick menu has less than 500 calories and contains at least three food groups.

Fast-Food Mexican Chains

When it comes to Mexican fast food, the best strategy is to keep it simple (*see* Weighing Your Options at Mexican Food Chains on page 168). Lower calorie meals include soft-shell tacos, bean burritos, and chili; for sides, look for baked tortilla chips and salsa. Hold the guacamole, cheese, and sour cream, or ask for these high-calorie extras on the side so kids can add just a dab to their meal. Order extra tomatoes, lettuce, chili peppers, and onions for crunch with a vitamin-rich punch.

WEIGHING YOUR OPTIONS AT MEXICAN FOOD CHAINS

Instead of:	Order:
Crispy shell meat or chicken taco	Grilled soft-shell meat or chicken taco
Chimichangas, quesadillas, tostadas, and chalupas	Fajitas, enchiladas, and tamales
Sour cream, guacamole, or cheese	Extra lettuce, tomatoes, and onions
Taco salad with shell	Veggie and bean burrito
Refried beans	Black beans
Nachos with cheese, guacamole, and sour cream	Baked chips and salsa
Chili con carne with cheese and sour cream	Chili con carne with onions

Quick-Pick Menu for Kids*

Soft-shell taco (beef or chicken), Mexican rice and salsa (small serving), a mango from home, and a carton of low-fat milk

or

Chili (large) with extra onions, a small salad with fat-free ranch dressing, baked taco chips and salsa, and water or a diet soft-drink

*Each Quick-Pick menu has less than 500 calories and contains at least three food groups.

FAST-FOOD ASIAN CHAINS

Although it's always been a popular carryout cuisine, Asian food is fairly new to the fast-food scene. Start with soup—most are broth-based and less than 100 calories per serving. Look for made-to-order stir-fry dishes and ask for them to be prepared with less oil and extra vegetables. Choose steamed brown rice instead of white rice or fried rice. Encourage kids to use chopsticks instead of a fork to slow down the pace of their eating. Finally, read the fortune, but skip the cookie. Who could predict that this tiny dessert would have 40 calories? *See* Weighing Your Options at Asian Food Chains for more ordering advice.

WEIGHING YOUR OPTIONS AT ASIAN FOOD CHAINS

Instead of:	Order:
Fried egg rolls, spare ribs, tempura	Egg drop soup, miso soup, steamed veggie spring rolls, or hot-and-sour soup
Battered or deep-fried dishes (sweet-and-sour pork, General Tso's chicken)	Stir-fried, steamed, roasted, or broiled entrées (shrimp lo mcin or chop suey)
Deep-fried tofu	Steamed or baked tofu
Coconut milk, sweet-and-sour sauce	Ponzu sauce, rice wine vinegar, wasabi, ginger, or low-sodium soy sauce
Fried rice	Steamed brown rice
Salads with crispy noodles, fried wontons, and regular dressing	Edamame (fresh soybeans), cucumber salad, stir-fried vegetables

Quick-Pick Menu for Kids*

Hot-and-sour soup, broccoli beef, brown rice, stir-fried veggies, and water or a diet soft drink

or

Egg drop soup, a steamed veggie spring roll, and kung pao chicken (hold the rice)

*Each Quick-Pick menu has less than 500 calories and contains at least three food groups.

How Does Your Kid's Fast-Food Meal Measure Up?

Take a few moments to review your child's or teen's fast-food habits. Start by reflecting back on a recent fast-food meal or snack. Write down what he or she ordered, including the portion size for each menu item. Then check the restaurant's Web site for the nutritional breakdown of each menu item and add this information to your record. To go a little farther, use the MyPlate information from Chapter 3 to list the food groups and the amounts from these groups next to each menu item.

Concession Stand Cuisine

Wherever kids hang out—movie theaters, amusement parks, sporting events, beaches, or pools—you'll find a concession stand. All the tips and strategies you've already learned for fast-food chains apply to the snack shacks, too. However, concession stands sell a few other treats, like cotton candy and buttered popcorn, that can sabotage your kid's weight (*see* Weighing Your Options at the Concession Stand).

WEIGHING YOUR OPTIONS AT THE CONCESSION STAND

Instead of:	Order:
Doughnut	Low-fat fruit muffin
Toaster pastries	Small bagel (or split a large one)
Sausage pizza	Cheese pizza
Hot dog	Small turkey sub
Potato chips	Baked chips or pretzels
French fries	Carrot sticks
Soft drink	100% fruit juice or low-fat milk
Sport drink	Water
Candy bar	Fruit cup
Ice cream bar	Frozen yogurt
Chocolate chip cookies	Animal crackers or graham crackers

Road Trip Eating Tips

When you're on the road, fast food is *not* your family's only option. If you know you're going to be out all day, pack a picnic of *Go for It* foods (*see* Chapter 3 for lists of these foods). Here are some tips and packing ideas for your kid's meals on the go:

- *Keep your cool.* Fill a cooler with healthy meal and snack choices, such as fresh fruit, fruit cups, packs of ready-to-eat raw veggies (buy prepackaged or make your own), low-fat cheese sticks, low-fat yogurt, peanut butter and low-fat crackers, water, premade sandwiches on whole grain bread (try lean turkey or ham and low-fat cheese), 100 percent juice, pretzels, animal crackers, and graham cracker sticks.
- *Bring water bottles.* Make sure everyone has their own water bottle to sip on the trip.
- *Refuel the car, not your kids, at gas stations.* The stores attached to most gas stations are stocked with high-calorie temptations such as candy bars, hot dogs, and soft drinks. When you gas up, keep the kids in the car and offer a snack from your cooler.
- *Stop at rest areas and stretch!* Steer kids away from vending areas, but let them get out of the car and move around. Many rest areas even offer playgrounds.

> **Parents Weigh In: Dinner Rescue Plan**
>
> After I started planning my dinners on the weekend, I couldn't believe how easy it was to cut back on fast food for my family.
> —TONYA, MOM OF TWO GIRLS

Fast-Casual Family Restaurant Review

In addition to fast-food chains, many busy families also frequently eat at fast-casual restaurants where somebody takes your meal order after you've been seated. When it comes to fat, calories, and sodium, fast casual restaurant cuisine can be a ticking time bomb. However, fast-casual restaurants seem to have a slight nutritional advantage over fast food because they carry many more items on their menus, including a number of lighter and healthier options. The key is to know which choices to order.

Whether you're dining at a national fast-casual chain or locally owned family restaurant, the following four steps can help you navigate through the menu and order a healthy meal for your child or teen:

- Prepare in advance a menu plan of attack.
- Stay on appetizer alert.
- Place your order with confidence.
- Ensure a happy ending.

Let's look at each of these steps in greater depth.

Step 1: Prepare in Advance a Menu Plan of Attack

- *Preview the menu.* Check out the menu on the restaurant's Web site before you go and ask everyone to preselect a lower calorie meal. When you arrive, simply bypass the reading of the menu and place your order immediately.
- *Keep an eye on the kid's menu.* Hamburgers, hot dogs, spaghetti and meatballs, fried chicken fingers, and macaroni and cheese—the typical kiddie menu is loaded with fat and calories! If there are no healthy items on the kid's menu, your best bet is for kids to share meals from the main menu.
- *Beware of all-you-can-eat deals.* Try to avoid eating at restaurants that offer unlimited portions. They may be a bargain price-wise, but not in terms of a healthy weight. When kids can eat without limits, they are more likely to overeat (*see* Chapter 6).
- *Curb kids' appetites.* About 30 minutes before you arrive at the restaurant, offer your child a healthy snack, such as an apple, baby carrots and low-fat dip, or a slice of whole grain toast with reduced-fat peanut butter. Being less hungry will help lower your kid's calorie count, and possibly your dinner bill.
- *Do a balancing act.* If you know that your kids will be eating out for dinner, make sure they eat a lighter breakfast or lunch that day.

Another balancing strategy is to get them to do a little extra physical activity, like riding their bikes or walking the dog, to burn off some of the calories they will consume.

Step 2: Stay on Appetizer Alert

- *Keep an eye on the bread basket.* Pass the basket around and let everyone take a piece of bread, then ask to have the basket removed but not refilled. Keep an eye, too, on how much butter and olive oil your kids slather on bread—these extra calories add up quickly.
- *Start with soup or salad.* To curb your child's appetite, order a salad or broth-based soup or an appetizer of crudités (raw vegetables). Go easy on the dressing and dips. One ladle of salad dressing holds about two tablespoons and provides about 150 calories.
- *Make a meal out of appetizers.* Downsize kids' portions by letting them order one or two appetizers as their main meal. Appetizer portions are smaller than entrées, and they usually cost less, too.

Step 3: Place Your Order with Confidence

- *Look for "light," "low-calorie," or "low-fat" options.* These Healthy Weight choices are typically featured in a special place on the menu. Many fast-casual chains have their own name and symbol for these light-bite dishes, too.
- *Read between the lines.* Scan the menu and look for word-clues to help you determine which foods are higher and which foods are lower in fat and calories (*see* Menu Language: The Good, the Bad, and the Salty on page 174).
- *Practice portion control.* Fast-casual portions can be big enough to feed a family of four! Ask for two plates so you can split dishes or have the kitchen put half in a take-away container before the meal (your child can enjoy the leftovers the next day).
- *Take it easy on the sauce.* Stay away from entrées with rich sauces such as alfredo, béchamel, carbonara, or pesto. These sauces are typically made with butter, heavy cream, cheese, or oil, and they can add hundreds of extra calories. Alternatively, encourage kids to

order the sauce on the side. They can dip their fork in and get a smaller amount.

- *Double-up the veggies.* Order an extra portion of steamed vegetables, such as green beans or asparagus, instead of white rice or fries.
- *Send it back!* If something is not prepared right and light like you ordered, speak up. Restaurant owners want satisfied, repeat customers.

MENU LANGUAGE: THE GOOD, THE BAD, AND THE SALTY

To find the foods with the least amount of calories, fat, and sodium on a menu, learn the language. Check the menu for word clues such as those listed below. Often, these descriptive terms can help you order healthier meals.

The Good (words that indicate fewer calories and less fat):

- Baked
- Steamed
- Poached
- Braised
- Grilled
- Roasted
- Broiled
- Lightly sautéed
- Stir-fried
- Cooked in its own juice

The Bad (terms that usually translate to more calories and fat):

- Au gratin or in cheese sauce
- Deep-fried
- Prime
- Batter-fried
- Double crust
- Rich
- Béarnaise
- Escalloped
- Sautéed
- Breaded
- French-fried
- Scalloped
- Buttered
- Hollandaise
- With gravy, mayonnaise, or cream sauce
- Creamed
- Marinated (in oil)
- Crispy
- Pan-fried
- Pastry

```
MENU LANGUAGE: THE GOOD,
THE BAD, AND THE SALTY (continued)
```

The Salty **(sodium lurks in each of these menu descriptions):**

- Barbecued
- Cured
- In broth

- Marinated
- Pickled
- Smoked

- Teriyaki
- With cocktail sauce
- With soy sauce

Step 4: Ensure a Happy Ending

- *Order a dessert for the table.* Spread the family love and calories around. Ask the waiter to bring *one* sweet treat and many forks. Pass the dessert around so that everyone can savor the flavor of their share.
- *Pick fruit.* Many fast-casual restaurants offer fruit cups, grapes, and cantaloupe wedges even if you don't see them on the dessert menu. Look at the breakfast menu to see whether fruit is available, or make a special request.
- *Let your angels eat angel food cake.* Angel food cake is very low in calories and fat. It tastes great plain or paired with fresh berries.

Healthy Eating, Healthy Weight—You're In Control!

■ *After talking with the RD, the Andersons decided it was time for the whole family to kick the fast-food habit. They made some goals and filled out a family contract:*

We, the Anderson Family, will work toward the following goal(s) over the next one or two weeks: (1) Sit down on Saturday afternoon and plan dinner menus for the up-coming week. (2) Make better choices when eating out at a fast-casual restaurant by discussing the menu ahead of time with the girls. (3) Pack a cooler with a healthy lunch and snacks for the tournament next weekend. When we have successfully made these a habit, we will reward ourselves with tickets to the women's college soccer game next month. Signed: Lauren, Lindsey, John, and Marge Anderson.

The parents now plan ahead for tournaments and pack a cooler with healthy sandwiches on whole grain bread, fresh fruits, low-fat yogurt, and bottled water. When they do eat out, the family goes to a fast-casual restaurant that features healthy dishes with less than 500 calories per serving. Every once in awhile, Lindsey enjoys a single fast-food burger, small fries, and a small soft-serve cone. Everyone in the family feels better, and Lindsey is at a healthier weight. She continues playing soccer and is looking forward to trying out for her twin sister's team next year. ■

When you're short on time and your family is starving, fast food is a logical option. But there's no need to trash healthy eating just because your kid's meal comes in a disposable bag. Kids can halt unwanted pounds by following *Healthy Eating, Healthy Weight Strategy #6: Slow down the fast food! Eat fast food less than once a week.*

Planning ahead, especially when your family's calendar is packed with activities, is key to tackling this strategy. Start by setting a few family goals together and write a family goal contract like the one featured at the end of Chapter 2. Here are a few examples of goals to get you off and running:

- Plan weekly dinner menus (*see* Chapters 10 and 11) on Saturday or Sunday afternoon.
- Pack healthy snacks for kids to eat after school or at athletic events, instead of hitting concession stands.
- When dining out, discuss menu options and decide what to order before you get out of the car.
- Skip the sausage or pepperoni and order a thin-crust cheese pizza with some vegetables. Or have prepackaged salad ready at home to serve with a cheese pizza.

At the end of the week, sit down together and review your progress toward your goals. Use a tracking record similar to the one at the end of Chapter 2 to measure your family's accomplishments and identify areas for improvement. And don't forget to celebrate your successes with nonfood rewards!

9

Healthy Eating, Healthy Weight Strategy #7: Sound the Alarm!

■ *6:15 A.M. It's time for 17-year-old Michael Sanchez to get up for school, but he hits the snooze button—10 more minutes of sleep seems more appealing than breakfast. He's never really hungry in the morning; plus, he's trying to drop a few pounds. Michael rationalizes, "I get plenty to eat all day long." He eats lunch at school, stops with his buddies at the food mart for snacks after school, eats dinner with his family, and wolfs down two bowls of cereal before going to bed. However, later that morning, Michael had a splitting headache and was having a hard time concentrating in algebra class. For the tenth time in the past few months, he went to see the school nurse, Ms. Chang. After talking with Michael about his morning routine, and all the benefits of eating breakfast every day, she recommended that he try* Healthy Eating, Healthy Weight Strategy #7: Sound the alarm! Eat breakfast every morning. ■

Daycare, school, work—for today's busy families, the morning rush hour is about more than traffic. Everyone is in a mad dash to finish homework, brush their hair and teeth, and pack lunches before racing out the door. Squeezing in a quick breakfast hardly seems worth the time. However, if your child or teen is a breakfast skipper, like our teenage friend Michael, it's time to sound the breakfast alarm. Breakfast is arguably the most important meal of the day and nobody should leave home without it. This chapter will help everyone in the family open their eyes to the importance of eating breakfast and how consistently eating the morning meal can help kids reach a healthy weight.

Breakfast of Healthy Weight Champions

Kids come up with all kinds of excuses as to why they should take a pass on breakfast— "Eating breakfast will make me gain weight!" "I'd rather sleep." "I'm not hungry when I wake up!"—but research clearly shows that breakfast eaters enjoy all kinds of benefits in terms of weight, health, and learning. On the other hand, skipping breakfast can be a nutritional nightmare. Because breakfast is so important, many schools serve it to hungry students who may not have been able to eat at home (*see* Smart Choice: The National School Breakfast Program). Let's take a closer look at each of the benefits breakfast has to offer.

SMART CHOICE: THE NATIONAL SCHOOL BREAKFAST PROGRAM

For over 40 years, the School Breakfast Program (SBP) has been helping millions of kids start their day with a healthy breakfast. SBP is a federally assisted meal program operating in more than 87,000 public and nonprofit schools and childcare facilities. The school's breakfast menus are available for free or at a reduced cost to qualifying students and must be limited in fat and saturated ("bad") fat and provide one-fourth of the Recommended Dietary Allowance (RDA) for protein, calcium, iron, vitamin A, vitamin C, and calories. The decisions about which specific foods to serve and how to prepare them are made by local school food authorities. To find out more about the SBP, visit the U.S. Department of Agriculture Food and Nutrition Service's School Breakfast Program Web page (*www.fns.usda.gov/cnd/breakfast*).

Breakfast and Weight

One of the biggest dieting myths is that eating breakfast will make kids gain weight. No evidence supports this belief. In fact, the opposite is true. Eating the morning meal can actually help both kids and adults maintain a healthy weight. Kids who eat breakfast tend to be thinner and have lower body mass indexes (BMI) than their breakfast-skipping counterparts (for more information on BMI, *see* Chapter 2). How can this be? There are a few possible explanations. First, eating breakfast seems to jump-start the body's calorie-burning system (metabolism) after a long night's sleep (hours in which no calories are consumed). Second, breakfast helps curb kids' appetites. Kids who eat breakfast are less likely to overeat and are more likely to exercise later in the day. In contrast, kids who skip breakfast usually make up for the calories—and then some—before the day's end and have less energy for physical activity.

Breakfast and Health

Kids who eat breakfast every day have a nutritional advantage over kids who don't eat it. For starters, breakfast eaters are more likely to likely to meet their daily MyPlate recommendations for food groups such as fruits and vegetables (*www.ChooseMyPlate.gov; see* Chapters 3 and 7) and get the 40-plus nutrients their growing bodies need. On average, breakfast contributes less than 20 percent of daily calories while delivering more than 30 percent of important nutrients such as calcium, iron, and B vitamins. In fact, studies show that breakfast skippers fall short on many important nutrients, including vitamins A, E, C, B-6, and B-12; folate; iron; calcium; phosphorus; magnesium; potassium; and dietary fiber (*see* Chapter 3). And, to make matters worse, kids rarely make up for nutrients missed at breakfast at other meals or snacks. Eating breakfast also benefits heart health as breakfast eaters tend to consume more fiber but less fat and cholesterol over the course of the day.

Breakfast and Learning

Is your kid looking for help to ace a quiz? Breakfast prepares children and teens to meet the challenges of learning. Kids who regularly eat a morning meal tend to perform better in school, often scoring higher on tests. While adults may condition themselves to overcome symptoms caused by breakfast skipping, children cannot. They experience the very real effects of short-term hunger, such as headaches, stomachaches, and low energy levels. Hunger often interferes with their learning by reducing concentration, problem-solving, and muscle coordination. Skipping breakfast is especially hard on young children because basic skills such as reading, writing, and arithmetic are often taught first thing in the morning.

Eating breakfast seems to improve kids' overall behavior in school. Those who eat breakfast are more likely to attend school whereas breakfast skippers tend to be tardy or absent from school more often and may need to leave class to visit the school nurse because of hunger pangs or other symptoms caused by breakfast skipping or skimping. Breakfast eaters report having more energy and tend to be in a better mood, which helps them participate in school overall.

Rise and Shine—It's Breakfast Time

Despite the proven benefits of eating breakfast, breakfast skipping is skyrocketing. In 1965, 5 percent of 11- to 14-year-olds and 12 percent of 15- to 18-year-olds skipped breakfast. Today, around 20 percent of 9- to 13-year-old children and 36 percent of 14- to 18-year-olds skip breakfast. Why are so many kids hopping out of bed and running on fumes instead of fuel? Two frequent excuses are they don't have time for breakfast and they're not hungry when they get up. The following sections provide some pointers to help families break these breakfast-skipping barriers. Also, remember to be a good role model—make breakfast a priority and eat it, too!

Beat-the-Clock Breakfast Tips

The following time-saving tips are guaranteed to help kids eat a healthy breakfast when they're in a hurry:

- *Give me five!* Reset the alarm clock so that everybody gets up five minutes earlier. The extra time will give kids the few minutes they need to eat a quick breakfast.

- *Get organized.* Each night before school, make sure that everyone's homework is completed and in their backpacks. Also, have kids decide what they want to wear and lay out their clothes before going to bed. Another time-saver is to pack lunches in the evening and keep them in the refrigerator to grab and go.
- *Ready, set, breakfast!* Get ready for breakfast before going to bed. Encourage kids to help you set the table or counter with glasses, dishes, and spoons. Setting out nonperishable breakfast foods such as boxes of cereal, whole wheat bread, and fresh fruit can trim minutes of morning prep time, too.
- *Tune out distractions.* Every minute counts! Turn off the TV and ask tweens and teens to stop texting and put away their cellphones.
- *Keep quick-to-fix foods on hand.* Stock up on healthy, ready-to-eat breakfast foods like instant oatmeal, whole grain cereal, reduced-fat granola bars, whole wheat frozen waffles, whole wheat bread and bagels, bananas, fresh berries, tomato juice, fat-free yogurt, low-fat milk, hard-boiled eggs, and peanut butter.
- *All for one and one for all.* Get up before your kids and make a large pot of oatmeal or a batch of buckwheat pancakes that are ready to eat as soon they enter the kitchen.
- *Divide and conquer.* Give everyone a breakfast responsibility. Somebody pours the milk, another person toasts bread, another scrambles the eggs. Make sure everybody takes turns helping with clean up, too.

Tips to Wake Up Your Kid's Appetite for Breakfast

When kids complain that they just can't eat in the morning because they're still groggy from waking up early or nothing sounds good to them, try some of these eye-opening breakfast strategies:

- *Start with a light bite.* At first, tantalize your kid's tastebuds with something small, such as an apple or slice of whole grain toast. As time passes, build up his or her appetite by adding other foods to balance the breakfast.

- *Consolidate breakfast choices.* Look for ways to get more food groups in a small volume of food. For example, offer kids a breakfast burrito of scrambled eggs and low-fat cheese wrapped in a whole wheat tortilla, or make a whole grain toaster waffle sandwich filled with peanut butter and sliced bananas.
- *Be a breakfast sipper.* Whip up a breakfast smoothie of berries, fat-free vanilla yogurt, and low-fat milk, and let kids drink their breakfast.
- *Learn to love leftovers.* Some kids don't like traditional breakfast foods. That's okay. Breakfast can be any food kids like, even a slice of pizza, a chicken or lean beef sandwich, or soup. Leftover macaroni and cheese heated in the microwave oven makes a fine breakfast.
- *Prepare a backpack breakfast.* Let kids start their breakfast meal at home and then eat more after they've headed out the door. Have your child or teen drink a glass of fat-free milk at home. Then pack a whole grain muffin or a bag of trail mix made with whole grain cereal and dried fruit in his or her backpack to enjoy on the bus or walk to school.
- *Eat breakfast at school.* Check whether your child's school offers breakfast either through the National School Breakfast Program or by selling a la carte items (available in some high schools). If a la carte choices are for sale, review them with your teen so he or she can opt for healthy breakfast foods instead of doughnuts, pastries, and other foods high in calories, fat, and added sugar.

Breakfast: A Healthy Way to Start a Kid's Day

Eating something for breakfast, even if it is simply a piece of toast, is better than eating nothing at all. On the other hand, breakfast is not a magic meal that will automatically help kids reach a healthy weight and stay energized. Eating too much for breakfast can contribute to unhealthy weight gain, and eating a breakfast high in sugar leads to a quick rise and fall of energy that brings on hunger pangs by mid-morning. The bottom line: Kids need to eat a nutritionally balanced breakfast every day if they want to reach and stay at a healthy weight.

What Does a Balanced Breakfast Look Like?

A nutritionally balanced breakfast contains a healthy mix of carbohydrates and protein, lots of calcium, and limited amounts of fat and added sugar.

CARBOHYDRATES

Carbohydrates are the body's main energy source, providing fuel that kids need to grow and play. Just as there are different types of gas for cars, there are different types of carbohydrates (starches, sugars, and fiber). The best sources of "carbs" for kids are whole grain foods like whole grain cereals or breads (*see* Whole Grain Bread: How to Pick a Winner). These foods provide vitamins and other nutrients as well as dietary fiber, which helps provide a feeling of fullness, aids in preventing constipation, and may lower cholesterol.

> **Kid's Weigh In:**
> **Bran—News to Me!**
>
> I never realized that bran cereals were not necessarily whole grain cereals. I guess it helps to check the food label.
> —BEN, AGE 17

As a general rule, choose whole grain carbs with at least three grams of fiber. When selecting a whole grain cereal, choose one with less than eight grams of sugar per serving. To find the grams of sugar in a packaged food, such as whole grain cereal, check the Nutrition Facts label. The grams of sugar in one serving are listed below Total Carbohydrate (note: four grams of sugar equals one teaspoon). For more information on the Nutrition Facts label, *see* Chapter 6.

PROTEIN

Children and teens need protein to help them grow, stay healthy, and fight off infections. Protein also provides energy, but it doesn't really kick in as a fuel source until after the carbs are used up. While most kids get enough protein, they don't necessarily get it at their breakfast meal. This is unfortunate because studies have repeatedly shown that protein-rich foods make meals more satisfying and seem to play a role in weight control. Although

WHOLE GRAIN BREAD: HOW TO PICK A WINNER

Congratulations! Your family wants to start eating whole grain bread. But how do you navigate the choices in the bread aisle and make the best buy? Here are a few tips to help you bring home bread that's a guaranteed whole grain winner.

- *Play the name game.* Check the front of the package for words such as "whole wheat" or "100% whole grain" listed by the name of the bread. To use these words on a label, the bread must be made with the "whole" grain, including the endosperm, germ, and bran. Refined bread, often called "wheat bread," is *not* whole grain bread because the germ and the bran (which provide fiber) were removed when the flour was processed (*see* Chapter 3).
- *Look for signs.* Some bread packages sport a 100% whole grain seal on the front of the package.
- *Don't let the color fool you.* Some manufacturers make bread brown by using coloring, so don't assume all brown breads are whole grain. On the other hand, you can now buy white whole wheat breads that have all the nutritional benefits of other whole grain breads.
- *Scan the ingredients list.* For a 100% whole grain bread, the whole grain (whole wheat, whole grain oats, whole grain barley, etc.) will be the first ingredient on the list.
- *Get the fiber facts.* Read the Nutrition Facts and select a whole grain bread that provides at least three grams of fiber per serving.

scientists aren't certain why, eating protein-rich foods seems to help stave off hunger. For a healthy weight, it's important to eat *lean* sources of protein (*see* Lean Eggs and Ham on page 186) because fat is high in calories and can be detrimental to heart health. Some leaner sources of protein include Canadian bacon; lean cuts of ham, turkey, and beef; eggs; reduced-fat peanut butter; nuts; and low-fat and fat-free varieties of milk and other dairy products such as cheese and yogurt.

LEAN EGGS AND HAM

When it comes to healthy eating for a healthy weight, it's hard to beat an egg. One large egg has about seven grams of protein but only 72 calories. Also, compared to meat, eggs are cheap—under a dollar for a half dozen. But eggs have been shunned for decades because of their high cholesterol content, which is all in the yolk. Fortunately, numerous studies have cracked the case and the egg's reputation has been cleared. Eggs are actually 25 percent lower in cholesterol than was originally thought (one large egg has 213 milligrams of cholesterol), and they're low in saturated fat (1.5 grams per large egg), which is the real culprit in raising blood cholesterol and clogging arteries.

How many eggs can kids eat? While the American Heart Association (AHA) advises adults to eat no more than three to four egg yolks a week, there are no formal recommendations for children. If your child or teen likes eggs, go ahead and let them eat them. Just be sure to prepare the eggs in healthy ways, such as boiled, scrambled with lean ham, or in omelets with low-fat cheese. Keep in mind that AHA does not advise any restrictions on egg whites. In recipes, you can substitute two egg whites for one large egg.

CALCIUM

Kids of all ages need calcium to help them grow taller and to help their bones become stronger. However, many kids don't come close to meeting their daily requirements for calcium, which amounts to 1,000 milligrams for 2- to 8-year-olds and 1,300 milligrams for 9- to 18-year-olds. (One cup of milk provides about 300 milligrams of calcium.) Studies have repeatedly found that kids who don't include milk or other calcium-rich foods, such as cheese and yogurt, at breakfast are not likely to meet their daily calcium requirements.

Healthy Eating, Healthy Weight *Breakfast Guidelines*

Breakfast should provide about one-fourth of a child's daily nutrient and calorie needs. What does this look like in terms of food? Here are some guidelines based on the daily recommendations of MyPlate *(www.Choose MyPlate.gov)* to help you and your family put together a *Healthy Eating, Healthy Weight* breakfast (*see* Chapter 3 for more information about MyPlate):

- Include at least one selection each from three or more different food groups, choosing portions that fit within the child's or teen's personalized MyPlate daily eating plan (see *Healthy Eating, Healthy Weight* Breakfast Picks for Kids).
- Eat a whole grain carbohydrate with at least three grams of fiber per serving.
- Include a lean protein food and a good source of calcium.
- Choose foods that are low in fat and contain less than eight grams of sugar per serving.

HEALTHY EATING, HEALTHY WEIGHT BREAKFAST PICKS FOR KIDS

Food Group	Healthy Weight Choices
Grains *1 serving = 1 ounce* *(1 slice of bread, 1 cup* *ready-to-eat cereal,* *½ cup cooked cereal)*	• Whole wheat bread • Whole grain bagel or English muffin • Whole grain waffles or pancakes • Whole grain cereal with less than 8 grams of sugar per serving • Oatmeal
Fruit *1 serving = 1 cup sliced* *fruit or fruit juice, ½ cup* *dried fruit, 1 piece of fruit* *about the size of a tennis ball*	• All fresh fruit! • Unsweetened applesauce • Fruit canned in natural juice • Unsweetened frozen fruit • 100% fruit juice

(continued)

HEALTHY EATING, HEALTHY WEIGHT
BREAKFAST PICKS FOR KIDS *(continued)*

Food Group	Healthy Weight Choices
Vegetables *1 serving = 1 cup raw or cooked veggies or vegetable juice*	• All vegetables!
Dairy foods *1 serving = 1 cup milk or yogurt, 1½ ounces natural cheese, 2 ounces processed cheese*	• Low-fat (1%) or fat-free (skim) milk • Plain low-fat or fat-free yogurt • Reduced-fat or fat-free cheese

Protein foods
*1 serving = 1 ounce lean meat,
1 egg, 1 tablespoon peanut butter,
½ ounce nuts or seeds*
	• Canadian bacon or lean ham
	• Turkey sausage or reduced-fat beef or
	  pork sausage
	• Reduced-fat peanut butter
	• Eggs: scrambled, boiled, poached,
	  or in omelets

Here's an example of a breakfast that meets all of the *Healthy Eating, Healthy Weight* breakfast guidelines: a whole grain English muffin with reduced-sugar jam, two scrambled eggs, one cup of blueberries, and one cup of fat-free milk. Let's run through the checklist:

- The breakfast contains at least three food groups: Grains (English muffin), Protein foods (eggs), Fruit (blueberries), and Dairy (milk).
- The English muffin is whole grain and provides at least three grams of fiber per serving.
- The scrambled eggs are a *lean* protein food.
- The milk provides calcium and protein.
- The fat content has been reduced by serving fat-free milk; the sugar has been limited by using reduced-sugar jam.

Breakfast Make Over

Whether your child or teen is headed to daycare, preschool, grade school, or high school, he or she needs to eat a *Healthy Eating, Healthy Weight* breakfast every day. Let's take a look at some breakfast meals that are popular with kids and give them a grade: A, B, C, D or F. What determines the grade? The *Healthy Eating, Healthy Weight* breakfast guidelines, of course! You'll also find extra-credit menu suggestions to help boost each breakfast's grade up to an A. Once you review the examples, try the same exercise with your child's or teen's breakfast—does it "make the grade"?

BREAKFAST EATEN BY A FOUR-YEAR-OLD PRESCHOOLER

- *Menu:* One cup of apple-cinnamon cream of wheat plus two teaspoons of sugar, and one cup of whole milk
- *Grade:* C
- *Pros:* This breakfast provides a good source of calcium and some protein by offering whole milk.
- *Cons:* This breakfast provides only two food groups: Grains (cream of wheat) and Dairy (milk). Cream of wheat is not whole grain, so the fiber content is low (less than three grams per serving). The fat content of the breakfast is high due to the whole milk. The breakfast also provides too much sugar—the apple-cinnamon cream of wheat is presweetened and more sugar was added.
- *Extra credit:* To boost the grade from a C to an A, serve the following breakfast, which meets all the *Healthy Eating, Healthy Weight* guidelines: one-half cup of old-fashioned oatmeal with diced apple, cinnamon, and one-half ounce of finely chopped pecans, plus one cup of low-fat (1%) milk.

BREAKFAST EATEN BY A FIFTH GRADER

- *Menu:* One cup of frosted wheat cereal (12 grams of sugar), one cup of low-fat (1%) milk, and one cup of calcium-fortified orange juice
- *Grade:* B
- *Pros:* The breakfast provides three food groups: Grains (cereal), Dairy Foods (milk), and Fruit (orange juice). The milk is low fat

and provides a lean source of protein with calcium. In addition, the orange juice provides even more calcium.

- *Cons:* The frosted wheat cereal is not whole grain and has no fiber; it's also a presweetened cereal with 12 grams of sugar.
- *Extra credit:* To boost the grade from a B to an A, serve the following breakfast, which meets all the *Healthy Eating, Healthy Weight* breakfast guidelines: one cup of whole grain oat flakes (six grams of sugar) with a sliced banana for added sweetness; one cup of low-fat milk.

Breakfast Eaten by a Teenager on the Way to High School

- *Menu:* Two chocolate-frosted doughnuts and a 12-ounce can of energy drink
- *Grade:* D
- *Pros:* At least this teen ate something for breakfast! Breakfast skipping would earn an F!
- *Cons:* This breakfast is basically a sugar and fat fest. It provides only one food group: Grains (doughnuts). It offers no whole grains, protein, or calcium.
- *Extra credit:* To boost the grade from a D to an A, serve the following breakfast, which meets all the *Healthy Eating, Healthy Weight* breakfast guidelines: one whole grain bagel with two tablespoons of reduced-fat peanut butter; one cup of sugar-free hot cocoa prepared with low-fat milk.

Breakfast Is Served!

The sooner kids eat, the sooner they break that all-night fast. Here some quick-pick breakfast ideas that meet the *Healthy Eating, Healthy Weight* breakfast guidelines:

- Make a smoothie by whirling low-fat milk, frozen strawberries, and a banana in a blender for three minutes, and pour into a glass or travel cup. Serve with a few graham crackers or, for a quick, out-the-door version, add bran to the smoothie.

- Pour some whole grain flakes and low-fat milk into a bowl or large mug and top with some raisins or almonds. Alternatively, top whole grain cereal with low-fat yogurt and your child's favorite fruit.
- Sandwich a few slices of banana between two halves of a toasted whole wheat bagel. Serve with a glass of low-fat milk.
- Toast whole grain frozen waffles and top with some fresh berries. Top with low-fat yogurt or serve with a glass of low-fat milk.
- Microwave a whole grain pancake or mix up a batch from scratch. Top with some pineapple rings and a small dab of maple syrup. Serve with low-fat yogurt.
- Make a quick parfait by layering low-fat yogurt with berries and some low-fat granola or whole grain cereal.
- Scramble eggs with low-fat cheese and green or red peppers.
- Sprinkle grated Monterey jack cheese over a corn tortilla and fold in half. Microwave for twenty seconds. Top with salsa.
- Anything goes as long as it meets the *Healthy Eating, Healthy Weight* breakfast guidelines. Kids can enjoy a sandwich made with lean meat, low-fat cheese, and whole grain bread, or toast a grilled cheese sandwich made with low-fat cheese, whole grain bread, and sliced tomato.
- Mix raisins or dried cranberries into unsweetened instant oatmeal and top with chopped walnuts.
- Stuff a whole wheat pita with hard-cooked egg, low-fat shredded cheese, and sliced cucumber slices or red peppers.
- Spread peanut butter on a whole wheat flour tortilla. Add a whole banana and roll it up.
- Toast a whole grain English muffin and top with lean ham and low-fat Swiss cheese. Enjoy with vegetable juice
- Mix low-fat yogurt, dried fruit, and nuts into leftover brown rice. Sprinkle with cinnamon.
- Serve a slice of whole grain veggie pizza with a glass of fat-free milk.
- Wrap deli turkey, a slice of low-fat cheese, and lettuce in a whole wheat tortilla.

A Few Words about Lunch

Although this chapter focuses on the benefits of eating breakfast, lunch is an important meal for kids, too. Like breakfast, lunch helps keep kids fueled and alert for the classroom as well as for their afterschool activities. What's on kids' trays or in their lunchbox can make or break their learning and affect their weight, too. Since the number of overweight kids has been on the rise, attention has turned toward schools and what they serve on their menus. Thanks to watchdog groups, legislation, and government campaigns, school lunches have improved—under the regulations of the National School Lunch Program, they are lighter and tastier and are available for free or at reduced cost to eligible students (for more information on this topic, visit the U.S. Department of Agriculture Food and Nutrition Service's National School Lunch Program Web page: *www.fns.usda.gov/cnd/lunch*).

> ### Parents Weigh In: Cafeteria Cuisine
>
> At my son's high school open house, I sampled low-fat pizza and tacos. They were delicious and my son had no idea they were healthy!
> —JODIE, MOM OF 16-YEAR-OLD MICHAEL (AND COAUTHOR OF THIS BOOK!)

Instead of purchasing a school lunch, many kids prefer to bring a brown-bag or lunchbox special from home. While homemade lunches do not need to meet the National School Lunch Program nutrition requirements, they do need to meet *your* standards. Here are some tips to make sure lunches pack a nutritional punch and are on target for your child's or teen's healthy weight goals:

- *Put them in the chef's seat.* When kids plan their lunches, they are most likely to eat them.
- *Make a specific plan for the week.* Take some time over the weekend to pack lunch items for each day.
- *Can the soda.* Have your child purchase low-fat milk at school or pack a bottle of water.

- *Change it up.* Keep lunches interesting by varying the contents. Go heavy on vegetables, fruits, and whole grains. Add some lean meats and low-fat cheeses.
- *Keep it cold.* Use an insulated lunch bag with an ice pack to keep cold foods safe.
- *Pack a lunch that's adventurous.* Try something out of the ordinary, like a tortilla wrap or a peanut butter sandwich cut into the shape of a heart.

Healthy Eating, Healthy Weight—You're In Control!

■ *When Michael talked with Ms. Chang, the school nurse, he realized that his headaches and sluggish feelings were probably linked to his skipping breakfast. Breakfast skipping could also explain why he felt so hungry by the late mornings and loaded up on snacks that were likely affecting his weight. Michael asked Ms. Chang some questions about the food served at school, and she encouraged him to talk with Mrs. Jones, the school foodservice manager, who happened to be a diet technician, registered (DTR). Mrs. Jones went over the breakfast and lunch menus with Michael and helped him select meals that were satisfying and lower in calories. She gave him a goal contract she uses and suggested he fill it out. Here's what he wrote:*

> *I, Michael Sanchez, will work toward the following goal(s) over the next one or two weeks: (1) Get up five minutes earlier and eat breakfast. (2) Add low-fat milk and whole grain cereal to the grocery list posted on the fridge at home. (3) Choose lunch from the healthy options suggested by Mrs. Jones. When I have successfully made these a habit, I will reward myself with a new poster for my room. Signed: Michael Sanchez.*

After he started eating breakfast and choosing healthier lunches at school, Michael felt more alert in algebra class—no more headaches or trips to the school nurse. After a few months, Michael noticed that his jeans were not so tight and, in fact, he had lost some weight. ■

Busy families are tempted these days to save time and skip breakfast. In the short term, this may seem like a good plan, but skipping breakfast can lead over the long term to all sorts of health, learning, and weight problems for kids. A smart way to manage your family's time and help your child or teen be a healthy weight is to follow *Healthy Eating, Healthy Weight Strategy #7: Sound the alarm! Eat breakfast every morning.*

To get started with this strategy, call everyone together for breakfast this weekend and come up with some goals that will help your family rise to the breakfast challenge. Complete a family goal contract to get the troops on board (*see* the sample form at the end of Chapter 2). Here are some suggestions to get you started:

- Have each family member set their alarm five minutes earlier to have time for breakfast.
- Pack lunches the night before and put them in the refrigerator so they are ready to go.
- Give each family member a "breakfast duty," like setting the table, popping the bread in the toaster, pouring the milk, or cleaning up.
- Select whole grain cereals with less than eight grams of sugar per serving.
- Sit down on the weekend and plan a few healthy breakfasts for the week by using the *Healthy Eating, Healthy Weight* breakfast guidelines in this chapter.

10

Healthy Eating, Healthy Weight Strategy #8: Come Together!

■ *After a check-up at Dr. Lewis's office, Mr. Perez was surprised to learn that he had type 2 diabetes and needed to lose weight. Over the past few years, Mr. Perez had gained over 30 pounds, which he attributes to his job. He and his wife both work in sales, so they travel a lot and work long hours. On weekends he tries to exercise. As far as meals go, he has no routine—he eats whatever he can find and rarely eats a home-cooked meal at the table with his wife and their son and daughter. Mr. Perez was greatly concerned when Dr. Lewis told him that type 2 diabetes runs in families and can affect kids as well as adults, especially if the children are overweight. Mr. Perez's grandfather and father had diabetes and were very heavy men. His wife's mother and two sisters have type 2 diabetes. Determined to prevent this disease from happening to his son and daughter, Mr. Perez asked Dr. Lewis for help. He recommended that the Perez family try* Healthy Eating, Healthy Weight Strategy #8: Come together! Eat family meals at least five times a week. ■

Warning! Home-cooked family dinners are on the endangered species list. Compared to years past, families spend 45 percent less time preparing food at home or eating meals together at the family table. As families cope with long workdays and evenings packed with homework and extracurricular activities, cooking a family meal is often the first thing to get squeezed out of the schedule. Instead, families opt for fast food or everyone heats something up in the microwave, grabs their plate, and heads off to the den or bedroom to watch their favorite TV program or catch up on e-mail. It's time to reverse this "heat, eat, and retreat" trend. Family meals need to make a comeback. Studies continue to show that the more kids eat dinner with their family, the more likely they are to be a healthy weight. Therefore, if your family is like the Perez family and needs help solving the family dinner dilemma, keep reading. This chapter will show you how to make dinnertime the centerpiece of your family life, and you'll learn the basics for shopping, cooking, and eating meals that contribute to a healthy weight.

The Magic of the Family Meal

Waving a magic wand won't make your child a healthy weight, but sharing home-cooked meals might do the trick. Research shows that kids who eat less than three meals a week with their family are more likely to be overweight or obese. In contrast, kids who eat family meals five or more times a week are more likely to be a healthy weight. In fact, the greater number of family meals, the greater the weight and health benefits—especially if those meals are home-cooked. Let's take a closer look at the power of the dinner hour.

Eat at Home and Save

A meal at home can save you time and money, and, if you do the cooking, it can cut your calorie budget in half. For starters, eating at home reduces time spent driving back and forth to restaurants and waiting for your order. Also, home-cooked meals typically cost much less than carryout or fast-food meals. However, the main advantage to preparing and eating meals at home is the calorie savings. When you make the meal, you can control how much butter, oil, sugar, and salt are added to food. Plus, eating at home lets you scale down portion sizes. For example, a plate of lasagna at a restaurant might provide 850 calories, 47 grams of fat, and 2,830 milligrams of sodium (salt). In comparison, a portion of a frozen lasagna is a healthier choice (1½ cups contains 495 calories, 30 grams of fat, and 765 milligrams of sodium), and a homemade version is best of all (1 cup has 265 calories, 9 grams of fat, and 595 milligrams of sodium).

Family Meals: Weighing the Benefits

A healthy weight isn't the only benefit that kids reap from family meals. Kids who sit down and eat regularly scheduled meals with their family have:

- *Better eating habits.* Kids who eat meals with their family tend to eat more fruits and vegetables and consume less fried food, soda, and saturated fat compared to those who do not eat regularly with their families. Kids who eat family meals also get more calcium, iron, fiber, and vitamins—all of which are important for kids' growing bodies. In addition, dinner routines established when kids are young seem to carry over to adulthood, which may lead to lifelong healthier eating habits.
- *Good grades.* Family meals seem to give kids an edge in the classroom. Children who share meals with their family most nights of the week tend to do better on tests and get higher grades, and they are less likely to miss school.
- *Positive relationships with their parents.* Family mealtimes promote parent-child communication. Children who eat with their parents tend to have a more advanced vocabulary than those who don't. Mealtimes also provide a time and place for in-depth talks, relaxation, and catching up on family news.
- *Greater self-esteem.* Teens who take part in regular family meals are less likely to smoke, drink alcohol, or use marijuana and other drugs. They also are less likely to feel depressed and tend to get along better with their parents.

Dinner: How to Just Do It!

When families are overscheduled with work, school, sports, and volunteering, the obstacles to getting dinner on the table each night can be daunting. Here are 10 tips to help you get dinner on the table five or more nights every week:

- *Make family meals a priority.* Issue a challenge: every family member must make a commitment to come to dinner and stick to it—sign a family contract if necessary (*see* the sample contract at the end of Chapter 2). Everyone may complain at first. However, if meals are pleasant, kids and adults will begin to value time together.

- *Strive for five meals a week.* Get out the family calendar and choose the five family dinner nights. If your family is currently overscheduled, you may need to work up to five meals a week. Start with just one or two meals a week and plan to limit future activities that conflict with family dinners.

- *Plan the menu before the meal.* Ask your kids to help plan the menus—this gives them an incentive to come to the table. Also, advance meal planning cuts out trips to fast-food chains and can save time, money, and calories. Find a spot in your kitchen (like the refrigerator door) to post the family dinner menu. You can also text menus to older family members.

- *Keep dinner simple: serve one main item.* Your kitchen is not a food court. Not everybody gets to eat their favorite meal each night, and you don't need to serve elaborate feasts. Instead, provide meals that are balanced with plenty of ingredients that help kids reach and maintain a healthy weight.

- *Cook fast but eat slowly.* When your time is limited, cut back on food prep while allowing ample time to enjoy the meal and each other's company. Set a beginning and ending time for the meal so that family members can plan accordingly. Eating slower helps prevent overeating, and kids will be more likely to leave the table full and satisfied.

- *Have realistic expectations about kids' eating habits.* Younger children often have a tough time sitting still and will only last a short time at the dinner table. Tweens and teens can have mood swings that make or break the time you all spend together. Understanding the stages kids go through can help you have positive family meals (*see* Family Meals with Growing Children on page 200).
- *Be prepared for the premeal madness.* The time just before dinner can be a challenge, especially for younger kids. You're busy and the little ones are hungry, crabby, and clingy. Make a simple healthy snack part of the routine. Set out baby carrots and fat-free ranch dip for hungry kids to nibble on. Also make a predinner activity box for younger kids that includes paper and crayons. They can draw pictures of daily activities to talk about during the meal.
- *Turn off cellphones and the TV.* Family meals are really about uninterrupted time together. Make it a rule: no texting or TV watching at the table. If there is a "must see" show that occurs during dinnertime, record it for later viewing (*see* Chapter 4 for more information on the benefits of limiting "screen time").
- *Keep conversation light and positive.* Make mealtime enjoyable so kids will treasure the ritual and look forward to it. Save discipline and arguments for later. Allow everyone a turn to talk, and if everyone wants to talk at once, borrow the "talking stick" idea from Native Americans. Only the person holding the stick (or other special item) can speak (*see* Table Talk on page 201).
- *Delegate responsibilities for prep and clean up.* Before meals, kids can set the table and help toss salads and pour milk (*see* How to Set a Table on page 202), and after eating they can help wash, dry, and put away the pots, pans, and dishes. Make a chore chart and take turns. Listen to music so chores go faster and are more pleasant.

FAMILY MEALS WITH GROWING CHILDREN

As children develop, their eating behavior evolves, too. If you're aware of the stages of development, you can help make family mealtime a positive experience for everyone. Here's what to expect when kids join you at the dinner table.

Toddlers:

- Are messy eaters just learning to use forks and spoons. Parents need to be ready to wipe up spills.
- Do best with finger foods.
- Eat only one to two tablespoon of food at a time. Appetites go up and down during the day. Parents do not need to worry.
- Say "no" to new foods. When parents ignore the "no" and just eat and enjoy the food, the toddler will begin to eat and enjoy it, too.
- Need a quiet time before meals to calm down.
- Learn new words from mealtime conversations.

Preschoolers:

- Are curious and ask "why."
- Like to help mix or stir food, make sandwiches, or clean fruits and vegetables.
- Like to eat foods they helped prepare.
- Eat best when surrounded by pleasant conversation.

6- to 12-Year-Olds:

- Generally eat well.
- Are cooperative.
- Can carry on a conversation.
- Are more willing to try new foods.
- Tend to want the foods they see advertised on TV.
- Enjoy cooking and eating simple foods they make.

FAMILY MEALS WITH GROWING CHILDREN
(continued)

Teenagers:

- Are learning how to be an adult and are trying different behaviors.
- Are able to handle some responsibility for preparing meals.
- Are prone to big swings in mood and eating jags.
- Eat foods eaten by friends.
- Need to have adults listen and talk with them.
- May complain about family mealtimes, but still need adult conversation and family meals.

Adapted from *Eat Together, Eat Better Tool Kit*. Washington State University, Cooperative Extension, the Nutrition Education Network of Washington, and US Department of Agriculture Food and Nutrition Service. *http://nutrition.wsu.edu/ebet/toolkit.html.*

TABLE TALK

Not sure what to talk about? Here are a few topics to help get the conversation started at your dinner table:

- What was the most fun thing you did at school today?
- Describe something new you learned today.
- What is your favorite thing to eat?
- What's the most delicious food on the table?
- If you could open a restaurant, what kind would it be?
- If you lived in a different time and place, where and when would you live?
- Who do you consider to be a hero?

HOW TO SET A TABLE

Knowing how to set a table and use the utensils helps children feel comfortable in social situations—now and in their future. Need a refresher on table-setting techniques? Use the following diagram to help your family set the table tonight!

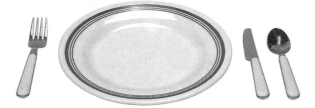

Healthy Eating Starts in the Kitchen

So, the kids want spaghetti for dinner. That seems easy enough until you reach into the pantry and—oops!—no noodles. Sound familiar? Whether you lack one ingredient or several, it's hard to make a home-cooked meal if you don't plan ahead. Let's get your kitchen into shape.

Parents Weigh In: Making a List and Checking It Twice

I can't believe how much planning weekly menus and making a grocery list helps me get a healthy dinner on the table five days a week.

—BARB, MOTHER OF THREE HUNGRY BOYS

Extreme Kitchen Make Over

Start your kitchen make over by purging your refrigerator and freezer of high-calorie, high-fat, and sugar-added foods and replacing them with healthier, lower calorie options (*see* How to Stock a *Healthy Eating, Healthy Weight* Refrigerator). In addition, spend some time reorganizing the fridge and freezer to encourage healthy food choices:

- *Reserve a shelf for healthy beverages.* Keep a pitcher of water with lemon slices in the refrigerator and stock up on fat-free and low-fat milk (*see* Chapter 5).

- *Divide your fridge in half.* On one side, keep all the food kids should eat *more often,* such as fruits, veggies, and fat-free yogurt. On the other side, keep the foods kids should eat *less often,* such as fruit juice and desserts (*see* Chapter 3).
- *Stock the shelves with healthy snacks and ready-to-eat produce.* Keep a cool stash of preportioned snacks such as small containers of fat-free, sugar-free pudding; string cheese; and baby carrots or apple slices with dip. Also stock up on precut containers of onion, bell peppers, and fruit to quickly add to sauces and stir-fry meals.
- *Fill the freezer with veggies.* Picked at the peak of freshness, frozen veggies are quick to heat and eat.

HOW TO STOCK A *HEALTHY EATING, HEALTHY WEIGHT* REFRIGERATOR

	Out with . . .	In with . . .
Grain products	Flour tortillas, white bread	*Whole grain* tortillas, bread, buns, bagels, and English muffins
Produce	Heads of lettuce	Ready-to-eat salad bags or fill-your-own bags from supermarket produce bins
Dairy foods	Full-fat yogurt, cheese, ricotta cheese; whole and reduced-fat (2%) milk	Low-fat or fat-free yogurt, reduced-fat cheese, low-fat or fat-free ricotta cheese, low-fat (1%) or fat-free (skim) milk
Deli meats	Salami, pepperoni, bologna, hot dogs, bacon, and sausages	Lean roast beef, ham, and turkey; fat-free 100% turkey or beef franks; extra-lean turkey bacon; lean smoked turkey sausage or kielbasa

(continued)

HOW TO STOCK A *HEALTHY EATING, HEALTHY WEIGHT* REFRIGERATOR (continued)

	Out with . . .	In with . . .
Frozen foods	Bulk ground beef or ground turkey, French fries	Individual lean ground beef or turkey patties and veggie burgers; cod fillets; chicken or turkey pieces; chicken or turkey tenders; boneless, skinless chicken or turkey breasts; bags of frozen vegetables such as chopped bell pepper, broccoli, corn, green beans, mixed vegetables, and chopped onion
Other	Stick butter or margarine, jelly, mayonnaise, sodas and sugar drinks, salad dressings	Tubs of soft *trans*-fat-free margarine; 100% fruit spreads and reduced-sugar or sugar-free jam; fat-free mayonnaise; bottled water; tomato juice; unsweetened iced tea; 100% fruit juice; fat-free salad dressings

After tackling the fridge, go through your pantry and cupboards and toss any expired cans of tuna or stale crackers. Donate higher calorie items to a food pantry. Fill the shelves with light and healthy ingredients for quick meals (*see* How to Stock a *Healthy Eating, Healthy Weight* Pantry). Here are some other pantry pointers to keep in mind:

- *Organize and prioritize.* Always store the lowest calorie foods in front and on the bottom (most accessible) shelves. For example, place whole grain crackers and cereal in front of baked goods so that kids will be more likely to make a healthy choice.
- *Beware of bulking up.* Buying in bulk may cost less, but it can lead to weight gain because the larger the package, the more kids eat

(*see* Chapter 6). Purchase single-serving portions or divide bulk containers of snacks yourself before storing them.

• *Stock the essentials.* Nonstick cooking spray is a pantry must—it doesn't add any calories and makes cleaning up much easier. Another Healthy Weight cooking essential? Canned tomatoes of every kind (sauce, paste, stewed, and in salsas)—they're perfect for adding to pastas, soups, stews, casseroles, and chilies.

HOW TO STOCK A *HEALTHY EATING, HEALTHY WEIGHT* PANTRY

	Out with . . .	In with . . .
Grain products	Sugary cereals (hot and cold), grits and cream of wheat, noodles, white rice, crackers, ready-to-bake mixes	Whole grain cereals with at least 3 grams of fiber and less than 8 grams of sugar per serving; oatmeal (regular and instant); whole grain pasta in a variety of shapes and sizes; brown rice; whole grain crackers; whole grain breadcrumbs; cornmeal; whole wheat flour
Canned goods	Fruits canned in syrup; vegetables marinated in oil; creamy or high-fat pasta sauce; fish and seafood canned in oil; soups; stews; broths	Fruits canned in natural juice or water; vegetables canned in water; beans (black, cannellini, garbanzo, kidney, and pinto); marinara and tomato pasta sauce; canned tomato products; water-packed clams,

(continued)

HOW TO STOCK A *HEALTHY EATING, HEALTHY WEIGHT* PANTRY *(continued)*

	Out with . . .	In with . . .
		crabmeat, salmon, and tuna; fat-free chicken, beef, and vegetable broths/stocks; reduced-fat creamed soups (broccoli, chicken, mushroom); reduced-fat soups (chicken noodle, minestrone, split pea, and tomato)
Nuts and nut butters	Peanut butter	Reduced-fat peanut butter; almonds; pecans; walnuts
Oils and seasonings	Vegetable oil; gravy and sauce mixes	Olive oil and canola oil; nonstick spray; seasonings such as basil, bay leaves, chili powder, cumin, dill, ginger, oregano, and paprika; vinegar; soy sauce

Make a List, Check It Twice

Congratulations! Your kitchen is reorganized and filled with healthy foods. Now how do you keep it that way? Develop a master list of your key ingredients and use it to keep inventory and shop for groceries. No more running out of the essentials or wandering up and down grocery aisles looking for something to make for dinner that night. Plus, shopping from a list makes it easier to resist deals on soft drinks and potato chips. Here are some tips to help you write a *Healthy Eating, Healthy Weight* shopping list for your family.

- *Organize by food groups.* Consider listing foods by categories based on MyPlate food groups (*see* Chapter 3). This will help ensure that your family meals include a mix of healthy foods.
- *Leave room for extras.* Add some type of catch-all grouping for extras such as condiments and spices. Also, make sure you have space for nonfood items that you may purchase at the grocery store, such as health and beauty products and cleaning supplies.
- *Fill in fundamentals.* If there are foods and other items that you must buy every week, give yourself a reminder by making them a permanent part of your list. For example, place fat-free milk under the Milk category heading or whole wheat bread under the Grain category. Then, if you need the item that week, just circle it.
- *Keep the list handy.* Develop a master list on your computer and print a copy each week. Keep the active list in a central location, like on the refrigerator door or in a kitchen drawer, where your family can add to it as needed.

Shopping Shortcuts

In addition to shopping from a list, here are some other shopping tips to help you save money *and* time:

- *Shop less and save.* Try to shop only once or twice a week. You'll spend less money on impulse items—and save time and transportation costs, too.
- *Buy groceries on a full stomach.* Try not to shop when you or your kids are hungry and more likely to be tempted by items that aren't on your list. Plus, your kids will be less likely to beg you for the candy at the checkout aisle.
- *Order groceries online.* Shopping for groceries online is affordable and handy. You can shop anytime day or night and have the food delivered at your convenience. You can even compare brands for

the best price, use coupons, and read the Nutrition Facts for products to get the healthiest buys.

What's for Dinner? 15 Ingredients = 5 Meals

Now that you have some healthy ingredients on hand, a delicious and nutritious dinner is only minutes away. As part of your kitchen make over, talk with your family and come up with a repertoire of five easy-to-make-meals that everyone enjoys. Then, to ensure you always have the ingredients for these meals on hand, make them permanent items on your master shopping list.

To help get your creative juice flowing, here are 15 go-to ingredients to stockpile:

- Brown rice
- Whole grain breadcrumbs
- Whole grain tortillas
- Whole wheat pasta
- Canned beans
- Canned tomatoes
- Canned tomato sauce or pizza sauce
- Frozen mixed vegetables
- Frozen chopped onions and bell peppers
- Reduced-fat cheddar cheese
- Eggs
- Low-fat chicken tenders
- Lean ground beef or ground turkey
- Frozen cod fillets
- Olive oil

With these ingredients in your fridge, freezer, and pantry, you'll have the staples to whip up the following five quick, healthy and tasty dinners (for recipes, *see* Chapter 11):

- *Quick Quesadilla* (recipe on page 257): whole grain tortilla, reduced-fat cheese

- *Pronto Pasta* (recipe on page 256): whole wheat pasta, tomato sauce, mixed vegetables, and reduced-fat cheese (meat is optional)
- *Go Fish!* (recipe on page 255): whole grain breadcrumbs, egg, cod fillets, and olive oil
- *Speedy Stir-Fry* (recipe on page 258): Brown rice, eggs, mixed vegetables, and olive oil (meat is optional)
- *Slow-Cooker Chili* (recipe on page 248): Canned stewed tomatoes, canned pizza sauce, canned beans, onions and green pepper, and ground turkey

Feel free to mix and match ingredients and add your own personal touches. Make the rest of the meal easy: slice up some fresh fruit, put whole wheat bread or rolls in a basket or toss together a salad, pour low-fat milk, and ring the dinner bell!

The Wonderful World of Recipes

So, when you're in a hurry and your family is hungry, what do you cook? In addition to the great-tasting, quick, and healthy recipes featured in Chapter 11, you can find inspiration for family meals in cookbooks and magazines and by searching the Web. Food products and grocery stores also offer recipes and you can download cellphone apps that give you a recipe and the shopping list, too.

Trying new recipes can be fun, but sometimes you may want to rely on established family favorites. Luckily, you can transform your family's favorite recipes into *Healthy Eating, Healthy Weight* dinner winners, by simply following these three easy steps:

- *Switch proportions or change ingredients.* In many baked goods, you can cut back on sugar by one-third and still enjoy good results. With sautéed foods or with food cooked in a small amount of oil, try using less cooking oil. Also, you can always substitute

> **Kids Weigh In:**
> **Dinner Tastes**
> **Great**
>
> We have been trying some new recipes at home. Home-cooked dinners taste so much better than fast food.
> —TOMMY, AGE 14

healthier alternatives for less-healthy ingredients (*see* Healthy Baking and Cooking Substitutions).

- *Modify food preparation.* With a little know-how, you can make simple changes in cooking techniques that require little or no extra time (*see* Culinary Lingo). For example, skim fat that collects on a stew or stock, scrub rather than peel fiber-rich potato skin, skip salt in cooking water, or oven-bake French fries rather than frying them.
- *Reduce portion sizes.* If a recipe is high in calories, fat, or sugar, make portions smaller. For example, reduce the amount of cheese sauce on a baked potato from one-fourth cup to two tablespoons, and add some steamed, chopped vegetables and herbs for flavor. To trick the eye so less looks like more, serve smaller portions on smaller plates.

Want to see these three steps in action? Check out Building a Healthier Lasagna Recipe (page 213). With nine simple changes, the recipe gets a fiber boost, while calories, fat, and sodium are cut way back.

HEALTHY BAKING AND COOKING SUBSTITUTIONS

Instead of . . .	Substitute . . .
1 cup cream	1 cup evaporated fat-free milk
1 cup butter, margarine, or oil	½ cup apple butter or applesauce
1 egg	2 egg whites or ¼ cup egg substitute
1 egg yolk	1 egg white
Pastry dough	Graham cracker crumb crust
Bacon	Lean turkey bacon, Canadian bacon, or lean ham
Ground beef	Extra-lean ground beef or ground turkey or chicken breast
Sausage	Lean ground turkey or 95% fat-free sausage

HEALTHY BAKING AND COOKING SUBSTITUTIONS *(continued)*

Instead of . . .	Substitute . . .
Sour cream	Fat-free sour cream
1 cup chocolate chips	¼–½ cup mini chocolate chips
Mayonnaise	Reduced-fat or fat-free mayonnaise
Salad dressing	Low-fat or fat-free dressing or homemade dressing made with less oil
Whole milk	Fat-free or low-fat milk
1 cup cream cheese	½ cup ricotta cheese pureed with ½ cup fat-free cream cheese
1 ounce unsweetened baking chocolate	3 tablespoons unsweetened cocoa powder + 1 tablespoon vegetable oil

Adapted from National Heart, Lung and Blood Institute. We Can! Fun Family Recipes & Tips. *www.nhlbi.nih.gov/health/public/heart/obesity/wecan/eat-right/fun-family-recipes.htm.*

CULINARY LINGO

To prepare a healthier family meal, adapt different cooking techniques. Discontinue deep-fat frying—it doubles or triples the calories, especially if the food is coated in breadcrumbs. Here are some potentially lower calorie cooking techniques to start using:

- *Boil:* to heat a liquid until bubbles break the surface. Boiling is a common way to cook foods such as pasta, sauces, and vegetables.
- *Bake:* to cook food in an oven. To ensure an accurate cooking temperature, use an oven thermometer. Foods that are commonly baked include seafood, meats and casseroles, vegetables, and baked goods.

(continued)

CULINARY LINGO *(continued)*

- *Broil:* to cook food directly under or above a very hot heat source (about 500 degrees Fahrenheit). Food can be broiled in an oven, directly under the gas or electric heat source, or on a barbecue grill (known as "charbroiling") directly over charcoal or gas heat. Foods that are typically broiled include meats, poultry, and seafood.
- *Grill:* to cook directly over a heat source on metal racks or rods or on a special grill pan. Meats, poultry, seafood, vegetables, and even some fruits grill beautifully.
- *Sauté or stir-fry:* to cook food quickly (for just a few minutes), in a small amount of fat, in a sauté pan or wok over direct heat. Foods that are commonly sautéed or stir-fried include meats, poultry, and vegetables.
- *Simmer:* to cook food gently in liquid at a temperature that is just below the boiling point so that tiny bubbles just begin to break the surface. Foods are typically brought to boil over high heat, and then the heat is reduced to simmer with a lid on the pan/pot to finish the cooking. Foods that are commonly simmered are sauces, rice and some other grains, and dried beans.

Adapted from National Heart, Lung, and Blood Institute. Keep the Beat: Deliciously Healthy Family Meals. *www.nhlbi.nih.gov/health/index.htm.*

BUILDING A HEALTHIER LASAGNA RECIPE

Here's how to revise a typical recipe for lasagna with nine *Healthy Updates* that save calories without losing taste.

Meaty Lasagna Recipe

Makes 6 servings (Healthy Update #1: *Change to 8 servings.*)

Ingredients:

16 ounces ground beef (*Healthy Update #2*: Substitute 12 ounces extra-lean ground sirloin beef.)

1 cup chopped onion

2 garlic cloves, minced

1 16-ounce jar pasta sauce (*Healthy Update #3*: Substitute fat-free pasta sauce.)

2 teaspoons dried basil

1 teaspoon dried oregano

6 dried lasagna noodles (*Healthy Update #4*: Substitute whole wheat lasagna noodles.)

1 beaten egg (*Healthy Update #5*: Substitute two beaten egg whites.)

1 15-ounce container ricotta cheese (*Healthy Update #6*: Substitute fat-free ricotta cheese.)

¼ cup grated parmesan cheese (*Healthy Update #7*: Substitute low-fat parmesan cheese.)

6 ounces shredded mozzarella cheese (*Healthy Update #8*: Substitute low-fat, part-skim mozzarella cheese.)

Directions:

Preheat oven to 350 degrees. For sauce, in a medium saucepan cook meat, onion, and garlic until meat is brown. Add pasta sauce, basil, and oregano, and simmer on low for 10 minutes. (*Healthy Update #9:* Drain fat from browned meat before adding sauce.) Meanwhile, cook noodles for 10 to 12 minutes or until tender but still firm. Drain noodles; rinse with cold water. Drain well. For filling, combine the egg, ricotta cheese, and parmesan cheese. Layer half of the cooked noodles in a 2-quart rectangular baking dish.

(continued)

BUILDING A HEALTHIER LASAGNA RECIPE
(continued)

Spread with half of the filling. Top with half of the meat sauce and half of the mozzarella cheese. Repeat layers. Bake for 30 to 35 minutes or until heated through. Let stand 10 minutes before serving.

How do the *Healthy Updates* affect nutrients and calories?

	Original Recipe	Revised Recipe	Savings
Calories	495	265	230
Protein	32.5 grams	27 grams	5.5 grams
Carbohydrates	25 grams	23 grams	2 grams
Fat	30 grams	9 grams	21 grams
Saturated fat	15 grams	4 grams	11 grams
Cholesterol	157 milligrams	40 milligrams	117 milligrams
Sodium	762 milligrams	595 milligrams	168 milligrams

Cooking Shortcuts

When serving family meals five or more times a week, it helps to know some cooking shortcuts. Here are some time-saving tips to help reduce your time in the kitchen to less than one hour:

- *Cook once, eat twice.* Prepare double batches of soups, stews, and casseroles. Eat one batch right away while freezing the other for a night when you need a quick meal. Use freezer-safe containers or resealable freezer bags, and label and date the packages so you know what's inside.
- *Serve planned-overs.* Transform last night's meatloaf into tonight's taco filling. Simply crumble the meat and stir-fry it with a dash of chili powder and cumin. Wrap it in a whole grain tortilla, top with vegetables and salsa, and olé!

- *Invest in family-sized cookware.* With a big, deep pot, you can make soup or baked beans from scratch, cook corn-on-the cob, or boil pasta noodles. With a large skillet, you can make pancakes, French toast, a big batch of scrambled eggs, or a vegetable stir-fry.
- *Consider a slow-cooker.* In the morning, toss some chicken, beans, vegetables, potatoes, and low-fat broth into a slow-cooker. Cover and cook all day on low heat. At dinnertime, you'll have a hot meal and your home will smell wonderful.

The Joy of Cooking with Kids

If you're caught between finding time to prepare meals and spending quality time with your kids, try cooking with them. The kitchen can be a fascinating place for kids to learn all kinds of fun things. An added bonus: your kids can be a big help to you, too. Read on to learn some of the things kids can learn in the kitchen.

Cooking with Preschoolers

Preschoolers can learn how to do the following while spending time with you in the kitchen:

- *Explore their senses.* Cooking lets kids get hands-on experience using all five of their senses. For example, by making pizza, they get to see the ingredients, hear the mixer whir, knead and stretch the dough, smell the pizza baking, and taste the pizza.
- *Build basic learning skills.* Cooking gives young ones a chance to practice skills they will need for school. They learn math by counting potatoes to peel, science by measuring flour, and reading by going over the recipe and following the directions.
- *Broaden their eating horizons.* Preschoolers are notoriously picky eaters (*see* Chapter 7), but cooking together gives them an opportunity to become more familiar with foods and increases the chances that they'll take a bite.

- *Boost self-confidence.* Cooking helps give kids a sense of accomplishment. They are proud to help out and enjoy their finished product. Kids get a thrill out of naming a recipe "Mike's Pizza" and telling others how they made it.

Cooking with School-Age Kids and Teens

School-age kids and teens can learn how to do the following by spending time with you in the kitchen:

- *Eat healthier for a healthy weight.* Cooking offers a perfect time to talk to your kids about nutrition. Planning a menu can become an opportunity to explain smart food choices and review the MyPlate food groups (*see* Chapter 3). As you're cooking, talk about why you're using fat-free yogurt or cutting the amount of sugar in half.
- *Apply what they learn in school to real life.* Your kitchen is really a learning lab where kids can brush up on their science, language, and math skills. For example, reading a recipe can help them learn how to add fractions and measure ingredients.
- *Share family traditions and conversation.* While baking Grandma's secret banana bread recipe together, you can share important information about cooking and Grandma herself, such as stories of her youth or how she taught you to make the recipe.
- *Become more responsible.* Cooking teaches responsibility in so many ways. Kids learn how to carefully use equipment such as mixers, knives, and ovens. They learn how to plan menus and follow recipes, and they discover what happens when you don't follow them. They can also learn how to clean up after themselves!

Culinary Kids: Getting Started

Before you grab an apron, here are few more things to consider to ensure that you and your child feel confident in the kitchen:

- *Choose the right time.* Ask kids to help you cook when you have time to explain what it is you want them to learn and do. Weekends work well for many families. Also, when cooking with little ones, make sure you choose a time when they're well rested. They'll pay more attention, and they'll be less likely to get frustrated.

- *Choose the right tasks.* Cooking is an art that needs to be mastered over time and with adult supervision. Make sure the cooking skills you're trying to teach are age-appropriate. Children as young as two years can help wipe tables, turn pages in cookbooks, rinse produce, and snap green beans or tear lettuce leaves. By the time they are ready to start school, children can also help stir batter, crack eggs, knead dough, measure ingredients, mash potatoes, peel oranges and bananas, toss salads, assemble pizzas and sandwiches, and set the table. Older kids can help plan menus and write grocery lists, and, over time, they can learn to use most kitchen equipment, including the stove and oven.
- *Choose the right recipes.* Younger kids may need to start out with basic recipes with less than five ingredients; teens may be ready to try more complex recipes.
- *Stress safety and sanitation.* As we've mentioned, kids of all ages need supervision when cooking. Make sure you set some kitchen ground rules with your kids, such as not to touch hot pans or knives and to keep fingers out of electric beaters. Go over these rules frequently. Also, when your child is helping you with food preparation, don't forget cleanliness. Teach kids to wash their hands using soap and warm running water before and after handling food or utensils.

What's Cooking?

Choosing a dinner theme is a great way to make your child's cooking experience and your family meals especially enjoyable. Kids get to use their imagination and create menus that are as much fun to make as they are to eat. To help your young chef get started, try the following themes created by the Eat Together, Eat Better Campaign of Washington State University, Cooperative Extension; the Nutrition Education Network of Washington; and US Department of Agriculture Food and Nutrition Service (*http://nutrition.wsu.edu/ebet/brochures/html*).

Spotlight Night

Birthdays are automatically special dinner nights. Between birthdays, make family members feel special with a family-member spotlight night. Celebrate the person by focusing on his or her interests. Have a special plate that the VIP (very important person) uses when in the spotlight. Let VIPs choose what to eat on their special nights.

Restaurant Night

Pretend you're at a restaurant. One person serves the food. Kids often think it is fun to be the waitperson and serve adults. Let them take your order and write it down on a notepad. Turn the lights off and eat by candlelight. If you have flowers, put them on the table.

Alphabet Night

If your family has elementary school–aged children, plan menus around a letter. For example, on "A" night, you could feature asparagus, apples, or apricots. Or use foods to help with reading. Write down all the foods used in the meal and use them as flashcards.

Game Night

Make individual pita pizzas (*see* page 260 for recipe), then play a game. Take turns choosing the game. The winner gets to lead the family in a fun exercise such as jumping jacks, push-ups, or hopping on one foot ten times.

Dinner and a Movie Night

Get a DVD and plan dinner around the movie. Try these movie themes and food:

- *South of the border:* Try kid-friendly Mexican foods: burritos, tacos, and chili.
- *Italian:* Serve meatballs and spaghetti or lasagna.
- *Asian:* Have stir-fried vegetables and rice, and eat with chopsticks.
- *African:* Try a bean dish. Africa has more types of beans than any other continent.

- *Old-time American:* Feature diner-style foods such as grilled cheese sandwiches or meatloaf and mashed potatoes.

GUEST NIGHT

Invite a grandparent or older neighbor over for dinner and serve one of your family's favorite meals. Ask the guest to talk about foods and meals they ate when they were kids.

Healthy Eating, Healthy Weight—You're In Control

■ *Mr. Perez and his wife joined forces and made the commitment with their kids to eat dinner together at least five times a week. At first the kids seemed a bit annoyed that they would have to cut their computer time, but it didn't take long to get everyone to pitch in. They even agreed to fill out a goal contract:*

> *We, the Perez Family, will work toward the following goals over the next one or two weeks: (1) Have everyone agree on five nights next week for family dinners. (2) Sit down on the weekend and plan next week's dinner menus and then make a grocery list to make sure we have all the ingredients. (3) Assign weekly dinner duties to each family member. When we have successfully made these a habit, we will reward ourselves with a day at the zoo. Signed: the Perez Family.*

After picking which nights would be family dinner nights, everyone marked the dates on their calendars. Mr. Perez visited the Academy of Nutrition and Dietetics Web site (www.eatright .org) to find a nearby registered dietitian. While on the Web site, he discovered a link to the Kids Eat Right site (www.kidseatright .org), which provides tips, menu plans, and recipes geared toward helping families shop, cook, and eat healthier. Within one month, the family was meeting their weekly family dinner goals. Mr. Perez's daughter really enjoys cooking and has accepted the responsibility of starting dinner on nights that her parents work late. Mr. Perez has already lost eight pounds and everyone feels healthier. They know there will be times when it seems difficult to juggle everyone's schedule and gather the family together, but they all agree to work hard to make it happen. ■

This chapter has explained how your family, like the Perez family, can follow *Healthy Eating, Healthy Weight Strategy #8: Come together! Eat family meals at least five times a week.* Family meals don't need to fancy feasts made entirely from scratch. All you need to get dinner on the table in a flash is a well-stocked kitchen, some healthy recipes, and help from your kids. Start by sitting down with your family and coming up with some goals to make family meals a reality. Once everyone agrees on the goals, make your own family goal contract (*see* the sample form at the end of Chapter 2). Here are a few suggestions for goals to get your plan in motion:

- Make a dinner-chore list to get every family member involved from preparation to clean-up.
- Make a list of healthy cooking essentials and take this list with you the next time you go grocery shopping. Make sure to include everything you will need for your weekly dinner menu.
- Turn off the TV and cellphones during dinner.
- Come up with five easy-to-make meals that every family member will enjoy.

Monitor your progress by filling out a tracking form like the one at the end of Chapter 2. Remember to keep the dinners simple and enjoy each other's company. Your family will make some lasting memories.

11

Healthy Eating, Healthy Weight Menus and Recipes

Planning meals ahead of time helps everyone in your family meet their *Healthy Eating, Healthy Weight* goals, but trying to come up with a repertoire of healthy menus and recipes can be tricky and time consuming. Luckily, this chapter can help jump-start your menu planning. You'll find three weeks' worth of sample menus for *Healthy Eating, Healthy Weight* family meals and snacks. Why three weeks? Because studies have shown that it takes at least three weeks to initiate a new behavior (*see* Chapter 2). You'll also find some of our families' favorite recipes—but more about that in a minute.

Menu Planning Made Easy

The suggested menus in this chapter are balanced and meet both the 2010 Dietary Guidelines for Americans and the MyPlate *(www.ChooseMyPlate .gov)* daily food plan recommendations (*see* Chapter 3). In other words, they include lots of whole grains, vegetables, and fruits, as well as fat-free or low-fat dairy products and lean protein foods. Averaged over each week, the menus provide all the recommended amounts of foods from each food group.

Here are some quick tips to help you customize the menus to your family's unique MyPlate daily food plans:

- Each menu includes breakfast, lunch, dinner, and one snack. However, some kids may need to eat two snacks a day to meet their daily nutrient needs, especially if they are going through a growth spurt or are very active. Chapter 3 has more snack ideas that you can add to these menus.
- Serving sizes are not included in the menus because they will vary according to your child's or teen's MyPlate daily food plan. (To find the right plan for your kid, visit the MyPlate Web site: *www.ChooseMyPlate.gov,* or *see* Chapter 3 and Appendixes A and B of this book.)

Really Good Recipes

For many of the items on the sample menus, we've provided delicious, easy-to-prepare recipes as well as nutrition information. (The nutrition information excludes ingredients listed as optional for the recipes.) Some of these are our own favorite recipes; others are from our favorite resources. Although we tested many recipes, we only included the ones that got a thumb's up from our kids. Try to get the whole family involved in preparing the recipes. Remember, when your kids are involved, they're more likely to try eating something new!

Three Weeks of Menus

Note: If you see an asterisk (*) next to a menu item, a recipe for that dish is included in this chapter.

Week 1: Day 1

Breakfast

Whole grain waffle
Reduced-sugar maple syrup
Frozen or fresh blueberries
Low-fat or fat-free milk

Lunch

Black bean salad*
Whole wheat pita chips
Orange slices
Low-fat or fat-free milk

Dinner

**Classic spaghetti
    and meatballs***
Tossed salad with low-fat
    Italian dressing
Roasted zucchini
Whole wheat Italian bread
Low-fat or fat-free milk

Snack

Baby carrots
Low-fat ranch dressing

Week 1: Day 2

Breakfast

Oatmeal with raisins
Sliced peaches
Low-fat or fat-free milk

Lunch

Turkey roll up: roll sliced turkey,
    low-fat cheese, beans,
    and salsa in a whole wheat tortilla
Cucumber slices
Mixed dried fruit
Low-fat or fat-free milk

Dinner

Go fish! Oven-fried cod*
Brown rice
Steamed broccoli
Frozen grapes
Low-fat or fat-free milk

Snack

Apple slices
Low-fat peanut butter

Week 1: Day 3

Breakfast

Breakfast burrito: scrambled
    egg, low-fat cheese,
    and mixed vegetables
    wrapped in a whole
    wheat tortilla
Mandarin orange slices
Low-fat or fat-free milk

Lunch

Grilled cheese sandwich: whole
    wheat bread, low-fat American
    cheese, tomato slice
Fruit salad
Low-fat or fat-free milk

Dinner

Lemon chicken*
Oven-roasted potatoes
Green beans sprinkled with
    low-fat parmesan cheese
Melon cubes
Low-fat or fat-free milk

Snack

Hummus dip
Whole wheat pita

Week 1: Day 4

Breakfast

Whole wheat English
    muffin
Canadian bacon
Pineapple rings
Low fat or fat-free milk

Lunch

Chicken tortilla soup*
Whole wheat crackers
Red bell pepper strips
Papaya
Low-fat or fat-free milk

Dinner

Speedy stir-fry*
Brown rice
Mango
Low-fat or fat-free milk

Snack

Salsa
Jicama sticks

....

Week 1: Day 5

....

Breakfast

Whole grain oat cereal

Banana slices

Low-fat or fat-free milk

Lunch

Tuna olé*

Tropical fruit salad

Low-fat or fat-free milk

Dinner

Turkey burgers*

Spinach salad

Watermelon slice

Low-fat or fat-free milk

Snack

Whole grain crackers

Tomato soup

....

Week 1: Day 6

....

Breakfast

Banana nut bread*

Cantaloupe cubes

Low-fat or fat-free milk

Lunch

Egg salad*

Whole wheat bread

Tomato slice

Plum

Low-fat or fat-free milk

Dinner

Quick quesdillas*

Mixed vegetables

Apricot pieces

Low-fat or fat-free milk

Snack

Graham crackers

Unsweetened applesauce

Week 1: Day 7

Breakfast

Cinnamon French toast*
Strawberries
Low-fat or fat-free milk

Lunch

Veggie pita pizza*
Apple slices
Low-fat or fat-free milk

Dinner

Cajun meatloaf*
Mashed potatoes
Steamed peas and carrots
Whole wheat dinner roll
Low-fat or fat-free milk

Snack

Plain popcorn sprinkled with
    parmesan cheese
Cranberry juice

Week 2: Day 1

Breakfast

Egg and veggie omelet
English muffin
Grapefruit chunks
Low-fat or fat-free milk

Lunch

Turkey sandwich: whole wheat
    bread, roasted deli turkey, sprouts,
    cucumber slices
Fresh peach
Low-fat or fat-free milk

Dinner

Liten-up lasagna*
Roasted eggplant
Garlic bread
Low-fat or fat-free milk

Snack

Berry blast smoothie*

....

Week 2: Day 2

....

Breakfast

Whole grain flakes

Dried cranberries

Sliced almonds

Low-fat or fat-free milk

Lunch

Bean tortilla roll-up*

Sugar snap peas

Fruit cocktail

Low-fat or fat-free milk

Dinner

Coo-chi chicken tenders*

Corn on the cob

Kiwi

Whole wheat dinner roll

Low-fat or fat-free milk

Snack

Banana split: banana (sliced
length-wise) topped with plain
low-fat frozen yogurt and
chopped nuts

....

Week 2: Day 3

....

Breakfast

Quick breakfast sandwich:
whole wheat English muffin,
poached egg, low-fat American
cheese

Apricot slices

Low-fat or fat-free milk

Lunch

Tuna bean smash*

Mixed vegetables

Diced peaches

Low-fat or fat-free milk

Dinner

Sliced ham

Baked sweet potatoes

Delicious greens*

Unsweetened applesauce

Whole grain dinner roll

Low-fat or fat-free milk

Snack

Celery sticks

Low-fat peanut butter

....

Week 2: Day 4

....

Breakfast

Low-fat cranberry muffin
Plain low-fat yogurt
Orange juice

Lunch

Ham and broccoli roll up*
Whole wheat breadstick
Tropical fruit salad
Low-fat or fat-free milk

Dinner

Hot and spicy fish*
Brown rice
Asparagus
Red grapes
Low-fat or fat-free milk

Snack

Small baked potato topped with
     broccoli and low-fat cheddar
     cheese

....

Week 2: Day 5

....

Breakfast

Whole grain toaster waffle
     topped with plain low-fat
     yogurt and sliced peaches
Low-fat or fat-free milk

Lunch

Chickpea salad*
Romaine lettuce leaves
Mandarin oranges
Pita chips
Low-fat or fat-free milk

Dinner

**Barbeque pork loin
     sandwiches***
Whole wheat hamburger bun
Corn on the cob
Watermelon wedges
Low-fat or fat-free milk

Snack

Whole grain tortilla chips
Low-fat cheese sticks
Pear slices

Week 2: Day 6

Breakfast

Egg and veggie pita*
Mixed fruit
Low-fat or fat-free milk

Lunch

Mac and cheese*
Steamed green beans
Red or green grapes
Low-fat or fat-free milk

Dinner

Slow-cooker chili*
Baby carrots
Tropical fruit salad
Garlic toast
Low-fat or fat-free milk

Snack

Frozen yogurt fruit cup*
Animal crackers

Week 2: Day 7

Breakfast

Whole wheat pancakes
Turkey sausage
Honeydew melon slices
Low-fat or fat-free milk

Lunch

Vegetable soup
Fresh pear
Whole grain breadstick
Low-fat or fat-free milk

Dinner

**Spicy southern barbecue
    chicken***
Baked potato wedges
Collard greens
Fresh melon
Low-fat or fat-free milk

Snack

Whole grain tortilla chips
Black bean salad*

Week 3: Day 1

Breakfast

Oatmeal
Fresh berries
Low-fat or fat-free milk

Lunch

Apple tuna sandwich: **apple tuna salad***, lettuce leaves, tomato slices, whole wheat bread
Avocado slice
Low-fat or fat-free milk

Dinner

Sloppy garden joes*
Steamed carrots
Pineapple wedge
Whole grain sandwich roll
Low-fat or fat-free milk

Snack

Trail mix: whole grain cereal, dried cranberries, chopped almonds, and sunflower seeds
100% grape juice

Week 3: Day 2

Breakfast

Whole wheat toast
Hard-boiled egg
Cantaloupe wedge
Low-fat or fat-free milk

Lunch

Chicken salad*
Mixed greens
Whole wheat dinner roll
Fresh pear
Low-fat or fat-free milk

Dinner

Jammin jambalaya*
Rice
Steamed zucchini
Mango
Low-fat or fat-free milk

Snack

Warm whole grain breadstick
Tomato sauce (for dipping)

....

Week 3: Day 3

....

Breakfast

Whole grain waffle
   topped with banana
   slices and cinnamon
Low-fat or fat-free milk

Lunch

Soft-shell beef taco: whole wheat
   tortilla, lean ground beef,
   salad greens, chopped tomatoes
Diced pineapple
Low-fat or fat-free milk

Dinner

Pronto pasta primavera*
Romaine and dark-green
   lettuce salad
Mixed fruit salad
Low-fat or fat-free milk

Snack

Mini sandwich: whole grain dinner
   roll, deli turkey, low-fat
   American cheese, dijon mustard

....

Week 3: Day 4

....

Breakfast

Whole wheat toast
Low-fat peanut butter
Pear slices
Low-fat or fat-free milk

Lunch

Chef salad: lettuce greens, diced
   ham, diced hard-boiled egg,
   tomatoes, low-fat salad dressing
Mandarin oranges
Whole wheat cracker
Low-fat or fat-free milk

Dinner

Grilled swordfish*
Orange couscous*
Steamed spinach
Sliced melon
Low-fat or fat-free milk

Snack

Chili popcorn*
100% grape juice

Week 3: Day 5

Breakfast

Whole grain oats
Frozen or fresh berries
Low-fat or fat-free milk

Lunch

Toasted mini whole grain bagel
Low-fat peanut butter
Sliced bananas
Jicama sticks
Low-fat or fat-free milk

Dinner

Thin-crust cheese and
  vegetable pizza (frozen
  or ordered from your
  favorite restaurant)
Raw vegetables (carrots,
  broccoli, cucumbers)
  with low-fat ranch
  dressing
**Fruit kabobs with
  fluffy fruit dip***
Low-fat or fat-free milk

Snack

Soft whole grain pretzel with
  mustard
Fruit cocktail

Week 3: Day 6

Breakfast

Whole wheat blueberry muffin*
Low-fat plain yogurt
Orange juice

Lunch

Pasta salad*
Low-fat string cheese
Strawberries
Low-fat or fat-free milk

Dinner

Grilled chicken breast
Baked sweet potato
Grilled vegetables
Whole wheat dinner roll
Low-fat or fat-free milk

Snack

Mixed fruit salad
Low-fat cottage cheese

Breakfast

Baked egg and cheese*
Fresh melon
Low-fat or fat-free milk

Lunch

Toasted turkey and cheese
   sandwich
Cucumber slices
Cherry tomatoes
Orange sections
Low-fat or fat-free milk

Dinner

Baked pork chops*
Oven-browned potatoes
Steamed broccoli
Diced apricots
Low-fat or fat-free milk

Snack

Grilled veggie wrap (use leftover
   veggies from the night before)
Water with a lemon slice

Family-Approved Recipes

Breakfast

· ·

Baked Egg and Cheese
· ·

Makes 4 servings

Ingredients:

1 teaspoon oil

6 eggs

½ cup fat-free milk

½ cup low-fat grated cheese

1 teaspoon garlic

1½ teaspoons oregano

Directions:

Preheat oven to 350 degrees. Put oil in a medium baking dish or small cake pan and heat in oven for 5 minutes. In a bowl, beat eggs. Mix in remaining ingredients. Pour into hot pan. Bake 20 minutes or until eggs are firm. Serve immediately.

> *Nutrition information per serving:* 144 calories, 8.8 g fat, 2.8 g saturated fat, 282 g cholesterol, 195 mg sodium, 3.2 g carbohydrate, 0.4 g dietary fiber, 13 g protein.
>
> Recipe from U.S. Department of Agriculture. The Healthy Family Guidebook. *www.nal.usda.gov/fsn/Loving/HealthyFamilyGuidebookEnglish.pdf.*

· ·

Banana Nut Bread
· ·

Makes 1 loaf (16 slices)

Ingredients:

1 cup mashed ripe bananas

⅓ cup fat-free milk

½ cup packed brown sugar

¼ cup margarine

1 egg

2 cups sifted all-purpose flour

1 teaspoon baking powder

½ teaspoon baking soda

½ teaspoon salt

½ cup chopped pecans or walnuts (optional)

Directions:

Preheat oven to 350 degrees. Lightly spray a 9×5-inch loaf pan with cooking spray. Stir together mashed bananas and milk; set aside. Cream brown sugar and margarine together until light. Beat in egg. Add banana mixture; beat well. Sift together flour, baking powder, baking soda, and salt; add all at once to liquid ingredients. Stir until well blended. Stir in nuts (optional) and pour in prepared pan. Bake 50 to 55 minutes or until toothpick inserted in center comes out clean. Cool 5 minutes in pan. Remove from pan and complete cooling on a wire rack before slicing.

> *Nutrition information per 1 slice: (without nuts):* 135 calories, 3.4 g fat, 0.7 g saturated fat, 14 mg cholesterol, 222 mg sodium, 24 g carbohydrate, 0.8 g dietary fiber, 3 g protein.

> Recipe adapted from National Heart, Lung, and Blood Institute. Stay Young at Heart: Cooking the Heart Healthy Way. *www.nhlbi.nih.gov/health/public/ heart/other/syah/index.htm.*

· ·

Cinnamon French Toast
· ·

Makes 6 servings

Ingredients:

2 large eggs

½ cup fat-free milk

½ teaspoon vanilla

1½ teaspoon ground cinnamon, or to taste

6 slices whole wheat bread

Cooking spray

Light pancake syrup or sliced fresh fruit (optional)

Directions:

Thoroughly mix eggs, milk, vanilla, and cinnamon. Dip both sides of the bread slices, one at a time, into egg mixture. Redip if necessary, until all of the egg mixture is absorbed into the bread. Spray a nonstick skillet with cooking spray. Heat over medium heat. Place dipped bread slices on heated skillet. Cook 2 to 3 minutes per side or until both sides are golden brown. Drizzle with pancake syrup or top with sliced fresh fruit (optional). Serve warm.

> *Nutrition information per serving (excluding syrup and fruit):* 123 calories, 2.3 g fat, 0.6 g saturated fat, 61 mg cholesterol, 189 mg sodium, 16.2 g carbohydrate, 2 g dietary fiber, 8.4 g protein.

Egg and Veggie Pita

Makes 4 servings

Ingredients:

4 large eggs

2 tablespoons low-fat milk

Cooking spray

2 whole grain pita pockets
 (cut in half)

½ cup low-fat shredded cheese

⅓ cup thinly sliced zucchini

⅓ cup thinly sliced red pepper

Directions:

Mix eggs and milk together in a bowl. Heat a small frying pan on stove. Lightly coat pan with cooking spray and pour in egg mixture. Cook for 2 to 3 minutes, stirring constantly. Place scrambled eggs in pita halves, and top with cheese and vegetables (you can also add vegetables to eggs while cooking).

Nutrition information per serving: 192 calories, 6 g fat, 2 g saturated fat, 183 mg cholesterol, 331.5 mg sodium, 20.7 g carbohydrate, 2.7 g dietary fiber, 13.5 g protein.

Whole Wheat Blueberry Muffins

Makes 12 muffins

Ingredients:

Cooking spray

1 cup whole wheat flour

¾ cup all-purpose flour

¼ cup firmly packed
 light brown sugar

1 tablespoon plus
 1 teaspoon baking powder

1 teaspoon ground cinnamon

½ teaspoon ground allspice

1 cup fat-free milk

2 tablespoons canola
 or vegetable oil

2 tablespoons unsweetened
 applesauce

1 egg, lightly beaten

1 cup fresh or frozen blueberries

Directions:

Preheat oven to 400 degrees. Lightly spray muffin tin with cooking spray. In a large bowl, combine flours, brown sugar, baking powder, cinnamon, and allspice. In another bowl, whisk together milk, oil, applesauce, and egg. Pour milk mixture into bowl with dry ingredients, stirring until just combined (do not overmix). Stir in blueberries. Spoon batter evenly into prepared muffin cups. Bake until tops are golden, 20 to 25 minutes.

> *Nutrition information per muffin:* 149 calories, 3.1 g fat, 0.3 g saturated fat, 17 mg cholesterol, 150 mg sodium, 24.9 g carbohydrate, 1.9 g dietary fiber, 6.4 g protein.

> Recipe adapted with permission from *Healthy Favorites: A Booklet Full of Healthy Tips and Recipes*. 2008. Published by Let's Go! *www.letsgo.org.*

Soups, Salads, and Sandwiches

....

Apple Tuna Salad
....

Makes 3 servings

Ingredients:

2 6-ounce cans unsalted tuna
   in water, drained
1 medium apple, chopped
1 celery stalk, peeled and chopped

¼ cup low-fat plain yogurt
1 teaspoon prepared mustard
1 teaspoon honey

Directions:

Combine all ingredients.

> *Nutrition information per serving:* 185 calories, 1.5 g fat, 0.5 g saturated fat, 36 mg cholesterol, 427 mg sodium, 12 g carbohydrate, 1.7 g dietary fiber, 30 g protein.

> Recipe from Centers for Disease Control and Prevention. Fruits and Veggies More Matters Web site. *http://apps.nccd.cdc.gov/dnparecipe/recipesearch.aspx.*

Barbeque Pork Sandwiches

Makes 6 servings (1 sandwich per serving)

Ingredients:

1 pound cooked pork
　　loin roast

1 cup barbecue sauce
　　(homemade or your
　　favorite low-sodium brand)

1 teaspoon olive oil

1 small onion, chopped

1 green pepper, chopped

6 whole wheat hamburger buns

Directions:

Slice the pork roast into sandwich-size slices. Place pork slices in a microwave-safe bowl; pour barbecue sauce over the pork. Cover bowl with plastic wrap, and microwave on a high setting for 3 minutes. Sauté the onion and pepper in the olive oil for 2 minutes or until tender. Place the vegetables and pork slices on a bun, and serve.

　　Time-saving tip: Pick up a precooked pork loin roast from your supermarket deli counter.

> *Nutrition information per serving with bun:* 378 calories, 13 g fat, 4.3 g saturated fat, 63 mg cholesterol, 329 mg sodium, 41 g carbohydrate, 4.2 g dietary fiber, 23 g protein.

Bean Tortilla Roll-Ups

Makes 6 servings

Ingredients:

1 tablespoon olive oil

¼ cup finely chopped green
　　onion

¼ cup finely diced ripe tomato

2 cups cooked kidney beans
　　or pinto beans (or a
　　16-ounce can, rinsed
　　and drained)

¼ teaspoon ground coriander

⅛ teaspoon ground cumin

½ cup tomato juice or sauce

Pinch of sugar

6 whole wheat flour tortillas

1 cup shredded, part-skim
　　mozzarella or cheddar cheese

Directions:

In a medium skillet, heat oil. Add green onion and cook over medium heat until softened, about 2 minutes. Add tomato and cook for 1 minute. Add beans and cook, stirring and mashing, until mixture is smooth. Stir in coriander and cumin. Gradually add tomato juice or sauce. Cook over low heat until mixture is thick, about 15 minutes. Add sugar and stir. Remove mixture from heat, and set aside. To assemble, place a tortilla on a plate. Spread 2 tablespoons of the bean mixture along one side, sprinkle with 1½ tablespoons cheese, and roll up tightly. (Tortillas can be eaten at room temperature or heated. To heat, preheat oven to 250 degrees. Place tortillas in a baking dish and heat for 10 to 15 minutes.)

Nutrition information per serving: 305 calories, 9 g fat, 10 mg cholesterol, 329 mg sodium, 39 g carbohydrate, 7.5 g dietary fiber, 14 g protein.

....

Black Bean Salad
....

Makes 8 servings

Ingredients:

1 16-ounce can black beans, drained

1 10-ounce can of whole-kernel corn, drained

½ green bell pepper, chopped

½ red bell pepper, chopped

2 green onions, chopped

1 tablespoon canola oil

2 tablespoons lime juice

1 tablespoon fresh cilantro

Directions:

Toss together all the ingredients except the cilantro. Generously sprinkle the salad with the cilantro. Cover and refrigerate at least 1 hour.

Nutrition information per serving: 80 calories, 2.5 g fat, 0.1 g saturated fat, 0 mg cholesterol, 378 mg sodium, 14.5 g carbohydrate, 4.1 g dietary fiber, 3 g protein.

Chicken Salad

Makes 6 servings

Ingredients:

¾ cup reduced-fat or fat-free
  mayonnaise
½ teaspoon ground ginger
3 cups roasted chicken, cubed
  (*time-saving tip:* use a
  deli-roasted chicken)

½ cup seedless red grapes,
  cut in half
1 cup celery, diced
⅓ cup sliced green onion
Chopped walnuts for garnish
  (optional)

Directions:

Combine mayonnaise, ginger, and chicken. Stir in the grapes, celery, and green onion. Cover and chill at least 1 hour. (The longer the salad chills, the better the flavor!) If desired, garnish with walnuts just before serving. Serve on a bed of mixed salad greens along with a slice of whole grain bread.

> *Nutrition information per serving (excluding walnuts, salad greens, and bread):* 173 calories, 6.9 g fat, 1.8 g saturated fat, 52.5 mg cholesterol, 311 mg sodium, 7.8 g carbohydrate, 0.7 g dietary fiber, 19.4 g protein.

Chicken Tortilla Soup

Makes 6 servings

Ingredients:

1 14½-ounce can low-sodium
  chicken broth
¾ cup water
1 cup medium chunky-style
  salsa
2 teaspoons chili powder
  or hot pepper seasoning
10 ounces cooked chicken
  breast, cut into strips
1 8½-ounce can no-salt-added
  corn, undrained

½ cup cooked dried black beans
  (or use no-salt-added, canned
  black beans), drained and
  rinsed
1 tablespoon fresh cilantro
  (optional)
1 cup crushed baked tortilla chips
¼ cup (2 ounces) shredded,
  reduced-fat Monterey Jack cheese

Directions:

Place all ingredients except the tortilla chips and cheese into a large sauce-pan and heat to boiling. Reduce heat to medium-low and cook covered for about 5 minutes. Stir in tortilla chips and cheese. Serve hot.

> *Nutrition information per serving:* 178 calories, 5.6 g fat, 2 g saturated fat, 26 mg cholesterol, 680 mg sodium, 43.4 g carbohydrate, 3 g dietary fiber, 12.5 g protein.

Chickpea Salad

Makes 6 servings

Ingredients:

1 cup cooked or canned chickpeas, drained and rinsed

3 tablespoons diced green bell pepper

2 tablespoons peeled, seeded, and diced cucumber

½ tablespoon chopped fresh parsley

½ cup diced tomato

3 tablespoons snipped fresh dill or ¼ teaspoon dried dill

½ tablespoon lemon juice

1 tablespoon olive oil

Salt and pepper to taste

Directions:

In a medium-size bowl, combine all ingredients. Refrigerate for several hours to allow flavors to blend. Serve the salad on romaine lettuce leaves or in whole wheat pita bread pockets. You can also puree the salad in a food processor to make a chickpea spread.

> *Nutrition information per serving:* 76 calories, 3 g fat, 0.5 g saturated fat, 0 mg cholesterol, 122 mg sodium, 11 g carbohydrate, 2 g dietary fiber, 2.5 g protein.

. . . .

Classic Egg Salad
. . . .

Makes 4 servings

Ingredients:

6 hard-boiled eggs, finely
   chopped
¼ cup reduced-fat
   mayonnaise
2 tablespoons minced onions
   (optional)

2 tablespoons minced celery
   (optional)
Salt and pepper to taste
Pinch of curry powder (optional)

Directions:

Combine all ingredients in a bowl and refrigerate until cold. Serve the egg salad on toasted whole grain bread with romaine lettuce.

Nutrition information per serving (excluding bread and romaine lettuce): 133 calories, 8 g fat, 2.5 g saturated fat, 319 mg cholesterol, 222 mg sodium, 4 g carbohydrate, 0.5 g dietary fiber. 9.5 g protein.

. . . .

Delicious Greens
. . . .

Makes 4 servings

Ingredients:

½ pound mustard or collard
   greens
2 cups shredded cabbage
1 tablespoon vegetable
   or olive oil

2 tablespoons minced garlic
1 chopped onion
1 tablespoon vinegar

Directions:

Rinse mustard or collard greens, remove stems, and tear in small pieces. In a large saucepan, boil 3 quarts water. Add greens, return to boil, and cook 3 minutes. Add cabbage and cook 1 minute. Drain in colander. Heat a large skillet over medium heat. Add oil and sauté garlic and onion until light brown, about 3 minutes. Add greens and cabbage mixture and vinegar, and cook briefly, about 3 minutes. Serve hot.

Nutrition information per serving: 81 calories, 3.9 g fat, 0.5 g saturated fat, 0 mg cholesterol, 12.5 mg sodium, 9.2 g carbohydrate, 2.1 g dietary fiber, 3.8 g protein.

Recipe from U.S. Department of Agriculture. The Healthy Family Guidebook. *www.nal.usda.gov/fsn/Loving/HealthyFamilyGuidebookEnglish.pdf.*

••

Ham and Broccoli Roll-Up
•••••••••••••••••••••••••••••••

Makes 3 to 4 servings

Ingredients:

2 10-ounce packages frozen broccoli spears	1 cup shredded, low-fat cheddar cheese (4 ounces)
1 tablespoon light margarine	½ teaspoon dry mustard
1 tablespoon flour	12 slices deli-style ham
1 cup fat-free milk	(approximately 5 ounces)

Directions:

Preheat oven to 350 degrees. Steam broccoli until slightly tender. Set aside. In a saucepan, melt margarine over low heat. Stir in flour and cook for 1 minute. Add milk, cheese, and dry mustard. Continue cooking over low heat, stirring until cheese has melted. Remove from stove. Place two slices of ham together, then place broccoli spears across the ham slices, roll up, and place seam-side down in an 11×8-inch baking dish. Continue until all ham and broccoli are used. Pour cheese sauce over ham roll-ups. Bake uncovered for 20 to 25 minutes.

Nutrition information per serving (recipe analyzed for 4 servings): 181 calories, 6.1 g fat, 2.1 g saturated fat, 22.8 mg cholesterol, 471 mg sodium, 13.4 g carbohydrate, 4.3 g dietary fiber, 19.3 g protein.

Recipe adapted with permission from *Healthy Favorites: A Booklet Full of Healthy Tips and Recipes.* 2008. Published by Let's Go! *www.letsgo.org.*

. . . .

Pasta Salad
. . . .

Makes 8 servings

Ingredients:

1 8-ounce package whole wheat
   spiral noodles

2 cups broccoli florets

2 cups sliced squash

1 cup bell pepper strips

1 cup halved cherry tomatoes

½ cup sliced green onions

1 cup fat-free Italian dressing

⅓ cup shredded low-fat
   parmesan cheese

Directions:

Cook pasta per package directions. Drain and pour into large bowl. Add vegetables and mix with dressing. Refrigerate. Sprinkle with parmesan cheese just before serving.

> *Nutrition information per serving:* 236 calories, 8.4 g fat, 1.4 g saturated fat, 4.6 mg cholesterol, 383 mg sodium, 34.7 g carbohydrate, 4.6 g dietary fiber, 9 g protein.

. . . .

Spinach Salad
. . . .

Makes 4 servings

Ingredients:

4 slices regular or turkey bacon
   (optional)

¼ cup cider vinegar

2 tablespoons olive oil

2 teaspoons yellow mustard
   seed (optional)

2 teaspoons minced fresh
   parsley

1 teaspoon grated onion

1 teaspoon sugar

1 large bunch young spinach,
   trimmed, washed, and dried
   (Shortcut: use a bagged spinach
   salad)

2 or 3 hard-boiled eggs, sliced into
   rounds

Directions:

Cook bacon (optional) in a skillet over medium-high heat until crisp. Drain on paper towel and crumble. In a jar or small bowl, make dressing by combining vinegar, oil, mustard seed, parsley, onion, and sugar and mixing well. Add spinach to a large bowl. Pour dressing over spinach and toss. Top with crumbled bacon and eggs. Serve immediately.

To make a warm spinach salad, simply heat the dressing until it is about to boil. Pour hot dressing over the spinach and toss. Add the bacon and eggs. Serve immediately.

Nutrition information per serving (excluding bacon): 160 calories, 12 g fat, 2.5 g saturated fat, 113 mg cholesterol, 246 mg sodium, 5 g carbohydrate, 2 g dietary fiber, 8 g protein.

Tuna Bean Smash

Makes 6 pieces (3×4 inches)

Ingredients:

3½ teaspoons olive oil

1 cup chopped mushrooms

2 tablespoons chopped sweet onion

½ medium tomato, chopped

1 clove garlic, peeled and minced

2¼ cup cooked white beans (or 1 19-ounce can), rinsed and drained

6½ ounces tuna canned in water, drained and flaked

1 tablespoon chopped parsley

½ cup shredded, reduced-fat Swiss cheese

2 tablespoons plain breadcrumbs or cracker crumbs

2 teaspoons margarine

Directions:

Preheat oven to 400 degrees. Oil an 8-inch-square baking dish with ½ teaspoon oil (or use cooking spray). In a small skillet, heat remaining 3 teaspoons oil. Add mushrooms and onion, and sauté over medium heat for 2 minutes, until softened. Add tomato and garlic. Continue cooking for 1 minute. Puree beans in a food processor. In a medium-size bowl, mix the sautéed vegetables with the beans, tuna, parsley, and cheese. Spread in baking dish. Sprinkle with breadcrumbs or cracker crumbs. Dot with margarine. Bake for 15 minutes or until crusty.

Nutrition information per serving: 201 calories, 5.9 g fat, 1.3 g saturated fat, 16 mg cholesterol, 173 mg sodium, 20 g carbohydrate, 7.5 g dietary fiber, 17 g protein.

Tuna Olé

Makes 6 servings

Ingredients:

6 whole wheat flour tortillas
1 12-ounce can tuna packed in water, drained
2 cups shredded iceberg lettuce
2 medium tomatoes, chopped
1 small onion, chopped
4 ounces grated, reduced-fat Monterey Jack or cheddar cheese
Taco sauce or fat-free sour cream (optional)

Directions:

Place 2 heaping tablespoons of tuna across the middle of each tortilla.
Add lettuce, tomatoes, onion, and cheese to each taco. Fold in half, and
serve with the taco sauce and sour cream (optional).

  Variation: Substitute low-fat refried-beans for tuna, and toss in a few
sliced black olives.

  Nutrition information per serving (excluding optional ingredients): 283 calories,
  8.9 g fat, 2.8 g saturated fat, 37.3 mg cholesterol, 551 mg sodium, 26.3 carbohydrate, 3 g dietary fiber, 22.8 g protein.

Main Dishes/Entrées

Baked Pork Chops

Makes 6 servings

Ingredients:

6 lean, center-cut pork chops
1 egg white
1 cup fat-free evaporated milk
¾ cup cornflake crumbs
¼ cup breadcrumbs
4 teaspoons paprika
2 teaspoons oregano

¾ teaspoon chili powder
½ teaspoon garlic powder
½ teaspoon ground black pepper
⅛ teaspoon cayenne pepper
½ teaspoon dry mustard
½ teaspoon table salt
Cooking spray

Directions:

Preheat oven to 375 degrees. Trim visible fat from pork chops. Beat together egg white and evaporated milk. Place pork chops in milk mixture, and let stand for 5 minutes, turning once. Meanwhile, mix together cornflake crumbs, breadcrumbs, spices, and salt. Spray cooking spray on a 13×9-inch baking sheet. Remove pork chops from milk mixture, and coat thoroughly with crumb mixture. Place pork chops on baking sheet, and bake for 20 minutes. Turn chops and bake for an additional 15 minutes until pork is fully cooked (to a minimum internal temperature of 160 degrees). Serve immediately.

> *Nutrition information per serving:* 216 calories, 8 g fat, 3 g saturated fat, 62 mg cholesterol, 346 mg sodium, 10 g carbohydrate, 1 g dietary fiber, 25 g protein.

> Recipe adapted from National Heart, Lung, and Blood Institute. Keep the Beat Recipes: Deliciously Healthy Dinners. *http://hp2010.nhlbihin.net/healthy eating/default.aspx.*

. . . .

Cajun Meatloaf
. . . .

Makes 10 servings

Ingredients:

1 tablespoon olive oil

3 green onions, trimmed and chopped

2 ribs celery, finely chopped

1 large onion, finely chopped

2 garlic cloves, finely chopped

½ green bell pepper, seeded and finely chopped

2½ tablespoons Cajun or Creole seasoning

½ tsp black pepper

2 tablespoons low-sodium Worcestershire sauce

2 pounds ground sirloin beef (extra lean)

1 pound ground turkey breast

4 large egg whites, lightly beaten

1 cup fine dry breadcrumbs

⅓ cup low-sodium tomato ketchup

½ teaspoon salt (optional)

Directions:

Preheat oven to 350 degrees. Heat oil in a large skillet over medium-high heat. Add the green onions, celery, onion, garlic, and bell pepper. Cook, stirring occasionally, until vegetables are nicely browned, about 10 minutes. Stir in Cajun or Creole seasoning, black pepper, and Worcestershire sauce. Cool to room temperature. Mix the ground beef, turkey, reserved vegetable mixture, egg whites, breadcrumbs, ketchup, and salt in a large bowl until well combined. Shape into two meatloaves and place them into 12×6-inch loaf pans. Bake 30 minutes. Increase oven temperature to 400 degrees. Bake until nicely browned, about 30 minutes. Cool in pan for 5 to 10 minutes before removing and slicing into thick slices.

Nutrition information per serving: 159 calories, 6.3 g fat, 1.4 g saturated fat, 32.8 mg cholesterol, 522 mg sodium, 13 g carbohydrate, 1.2 g dietary fiber, 12 g protein.

Slow-Cooker Chili

Makes 8 servings

Ingredients:

1 tablespoon olive oil

1 cup chopped onion

2 garlic cloves, minced

1½ pounds ground turkey

1 15-ounce can black beans, drained and rinsed

1 14½-ounce can low-sodium diced tomatoes with chilies

1 15-ounce can pizza sauce

1 10.75-ounce can reduced-sodium tomato soup

2 tablespoons chili powder

1 tablespoon reduced-sodium Worcestershire sauce

¼ teaspoon ground pepper

Directions:

Heat oil in a large pan over medium-high heat. Add onion and garlic. Cook about 2 minutes until golden brown. Add turkey; cook until broken up and browned, about 5 minutes. Transfer turkey mixture to a slow-cooker. Stir in the rest of the ingredients. Cook on low heat for about 8 hours or on high heat for 4 hours.

> *Nutrition information per serving:* 297 calories, 10.8 g fat, 2.6 g saturated fat, 63 mg cholesterol, 213 mg sodium, 26 g carbohydrate, 7 g dietary fiber, 23.6 g protein.

Coo-Chi Chicken Tenders

Makes 6 servings

Ingredients:

1 pound chicken tenders
¾ teaspoon garlic powder
2 teaspoons curry powder, divided in half
1 tablespoon olive oil

1 14-ounce can low-sodium chicken broth
1 16-ounce package of mixed chopped vegetables (available in the produce department)
1 cup uncooked couscous

Directions:

Place chicken in a medium bowl. Sprinkle with the garlic powder and 1 teaspoon curry powder; toss to coat. Heat oil in a large, deep skillet over medium-high heat until hot. Add the chicken to the skillet, and stir-fry for about 5 minutes or until the chicken is no longer pink in the center. Transfer the chicken to a plate, and set aside. Add the broth, mixed vegetables, and remaining curry powder to the skillet, and bring to a boil over high heat. Cover with the skillet lid, and boil for about 2 minutes. Stir in the couscous, and top with the chicken. Cover and remove from heat. Let stand for 5 minutes or until liquid is absorbed.

Variations: For a sweeter flavor, toss in a few raisins with broth and vegetables. Reduce the curry powder to 1 teaspoon for a milder dish.

> *Nutrition information per serving:* 411 calories, 15 g fat, 3 g saturated fat, 29 mg cholesterol, 368 mg sodium, 50 g carbohydrate, 5.6 g dietary fiber, 19 g protein.

Classic Spaghetti and Meatballs

Makes 6 servings

Ingredients:

1½ pounds ground turkey breast

2 egg whites, lightly beaten

¼ cup water

½ teaspoon dried basil

¼ teaspoon black pepper

½ cup breadcrumbs

8 ounces whole wheat spaghetti

1 15-ounce jar of your
  favorite marinara sauce

Directions:

Preheat oven to 375 degrees. In a large bowl, combine the ground turkey, egg whites, water, basil, black pepper, and breadcrumbs. Shape into about thirty 1-inch meatballs. Place ½ inch apart on foil-lined baking sheets, and bake for about 20 minutes. (The foil is for easy cleanup!) To make the spaghetti, boil the noodles in a large pot according to the package directions. Heat the marinara sauce in a large saucepan on the top of the stove. Drain the spaghetti, and top with the sauce and meatballs.

> *Nutrition information per serving:* 352 calories, 4 g fat, 1 g saturated fat, 76 mg cholesterol, 424 mg sodium, 44 g carbohydrate, 7 g dietary fiber, 36 g protein.

Grilled Swordfish

Makes 4 servings

Ingredients:

2 tablespoons reduced-sodium
  soy sauce

2 tablespoons orange juice

1 tablespoon olive oil

1 tablespoon tomato paste

1 tablespoon fresh parsley,
  chopped

1 garlic clove, minced

½ teaspoon dried oregano

¼ teaspoon black pepper

1 pound swordfish steaks

Directions:

Mix together all ingredients, except the fish, to make a marinade. Arrange fish in a single layer in a large dish and pour marinade over fish. Cover the dish with foil or plastic wrap and refrigerate for 30 minutes. Turn fish over, and marinate for another 30 minutes in the refrigerator. Discard excess marinade immediately. Grill fish for 5 minutes on each side.

Fish switch: You can use tuna or halibut in place of the swordfish.

Nutrition information per serving: 200 calories, 8 g fat, 1.5 g saturated fat, 41 mg cholesterol, 323 mg sodium, 2.5 g carbohydrate, 0.5 g dietary fiber, 22 g protein.

Hot and Spicy Fish

Makes 4 servings

Ingredients:

1 pound white fish fillets, fresh or frozen (thaw if using frozen fish)

¼ teaspoon paprika

¼ teaspoon garlic powder

¼ teaspoon onion powder

⅛ teaspoon pepper

⅛ teaspoon oregano

⅛ teaspoon thyme

1 tablespoon lemon juice

1½ tablespoons margarine, melted

Directions:

Preheat oven to 350 degrees. Separate fish into four fillets or pieces. Place fish on an ungreased 13×9×2-inch baking sheet. Combine paprika, garlic powder, onion powder, pepper, oregano, and thyme in a small bowl. Sprinkle seasoning mixture and lemon juice evenly over fish. Drizzle margarine evenly over fish. Bake until fish flakes easily with a fork, about 20 to 25 minutes.

Nutrition information per serving: 184 calories, 9.7 g fat, 1.6 g saturated fat, 69.8 mg cholesterol, 92.2 mg sodium, 0.8 g carbohydrate, 0.1 g dietary fiber, 22.3 g protein.

Recipe adapted from U.S. Department of Agriculture Food and Nutrition Service. Eat Smart Play Hard Healthy Lifestyle! Web site. *www.fns.usda.gov /eatsmartplayhardhealthylifestyle.*

Jammin' Jambalaya

Makes 4 servings

Ingredients:

1 teaspoon olive oil

1 medium onion, chopped

1 medium green bell pepper, chopped

1 14-ounce can low-sodium, stewed Italian-style tomatoes, undrained

1 12-ounce package frozen, ready-to-cook medium shrimp, thawed and drained

8 ounces reduced-fat, fully cooked turkey sausage, sliced and quartered

1 teaspoon dried Italian seasoning

¼ teaspoon hot pepper sauce (optional)

2 cups cooked brown rice

Directions:

Heat oil in a large, nonstick skillet over medium-high heat until hot. Add the onion and bell pepper; cook until crisp yet tender, stirring occasionally. Add all remaining ingredients except the rice. Bring to a boil. Reduce the heat, and simmer about 5 minutes or until the shrimp turns pink, stirring occasionally. Stir in the rice. Continue cooking until the liquid is almost absorbed and the rice is thoroughly heated.

Fish switch: You can use scallops, clams, or lobster in place of the shrimp.

Nutrition information per serving: 340 calories, 8.5 g fat, 2.2 g saturated fat, 156 mg cholesterol, 505 mg sodium, 36 g carbohydrate, 4.5 g dietary fiber, 26 g protein.

Liten-up Lasagna

Makes 8 servings

Ingredients:

12 ounces extra-lean ground sirloin beef

1 cup chopped onion

2 garlic cloves, minced

6 dried whole grain lasagna noodles

1 16-ounce jar fat-free, reduced-sodium pasta sauce

2 large egg whites, beaten

2 teaspoons dried basil

1 teaspoon dried oregano

1 15-ounce container fat-free
 ricotta cheese

¼ cup grated, reduced-fat
 parmesan cheese

6 ounces shredded, low-fat/
 part-skim mozzarella cheese

Directions:

For sauce, in a medium saucepan cook beef, onion, and garlic until beef is brown. Drain and discard fat from mixture. Add pasta sauce, basil, and oregano, and simmer on low for 10 minutes. Meanwhile, cook noodles for 10 to 12 minutes or until tender but still firm. Drain noodles, rinse with cold water. Drain well. Make filling by combining the egg whites, ricotta cheese, and parmesan cheese. Layer half the cooked noodles in a 2-quart rectangular baking dish. Spread with half the ricotta filling. Top with half the meat sauce and half the mozzarella cheese. Repeat layers. Bake in oven for 30 to 35 minutes or until heated through and bubbling. Let stand 10 minutes before serving.

> *Nutrition information per serving:* 265 calories, 9 g fat, 4 g saturated fat, 40 mg cholesterol, 319 mg sodium, 23 g carbohydrate, 3.5 g dietary fiber, 27 g protein.

Lemon Chicken

Makes 6 servings

Ingredients:

¼ cup olive oil

¾ cup lemon juice

2 tablespoons oregano

2 tablespoon dried thyme

2 teaspoons fresh garlic,
 chopped

8 to 10 boneless, skinless
 chicken thighs

Directions:

Make marinade by combining all ingredients except chicken. Place chicken in a single layer in a dish. Add marinade. Cover dish with foil or plastic wrap and marinate chicken for 20 minutes in the refrigerator. Preheat oven to 350 degrees. Place chicken and marinade in an 8½×11-inch baking dish. Bake uncovered 45 minutes (to a minimum internal temperature of 165 degrees). Serve immediately.

> *Nutrition information per serving:* 261 calories, 19 g fat, 4.4 g saturated fat, 72 mg cholesterol, 65.3 mg sodium, 2.8 g carbohydrate, 0.7 g dietary fiber, 19.6 g protein.

Mac and Cheese

Makes 6 servings

Ingredients:

Nonstick cooking spray
2 cups whole wheat macaroni, uncooked
2 egg whites
2 cups shredded, low-fat or reduced-fat cheddar cheese
1 cup part-skim ricotta cheese

½ cup fat-free sour cream
½ cup fat-free milk
½ teaspoon salt (optional)
½ teaspoon black pepper
¼ cup dry breadcrumbs
½ teaspoon paprika

Directions:

Preheat oven to 350 degrees. Spray a 2-quart casserole dish with nonstick cooking spray. In a saucepan, cook the macaroni according to the package instructions. When cooked, remove from heat, and drain in a strainer. In a small bowl, beat the egg whites with a fork. Combine the egg whites, cheddar and ricotta cheeses, sour cream, milk, salt (optional), and pepper in the casserole dish. Stir in the drained macaroni. Sprinkle the casserole with breadcrumbs and paprika. Cover and bake 30 minutes. Uncover and bake for an additional 5 minutes.

> *Nutrition information per serving:* 287 calories, 7 g fat, 4 g saturated fat, 23 mg cholesterol, 377 mg sodium, 36 g carbohydrate, 3 g dietary fiber, 22 g protein.

Orange Couscous

Makes 4 servings

Ingredients:

1¼ cup low-sodium chicken broth

2 tablespoons raisins

1 cup whole wheat couscous

1 tablespoon fresh mint, rinsed, dried, and chopped (or 1 teaspoon dried mint)

1 tablespoon unsalted sliced almonds

Zest of 1 medium orange (rinse orange before grating the rind)

Directions:

Combine chicken broth and raisins in a small saucepan. Bring to boil over high heat. Add couscous, and return to boil. Cover and remove from heat. Let the saucepan stand for 5 minutes, until the couscous has absorbed all the broth. Meanwhile, toast almonds in the toaster oven on a foil-lined tray for about 5 minutes, or until golden brown. Remove the lid and fluff the couscous with a fork. Gently mix in the mint, almonds, and orange zest. Serve immediately.

> *Nutrition information per serving:* 141 calories, 2 g fat, 0 g saturated fat, 0 mg cholesterol, 24 mg sodium, 28 g carbohydrate, 4 g dietary fiber, 6 g protein.

Go Fish! Oven-Fried Cod

Makes 4 servings

Ingredients:

1 cup whole grain breadcrumbs

¼ cup grated parmesan cheese

1 teaspoon grated lemon rind

¼ teaspoon black pepper

Nonstick cooking spray

1 tablespoon canola oil

1 pound cod fillets

Salt (optional)

2 egg whites

¼ cup fat-free milk

Directions:

Combine breadcrumbs, parmesan cheese, lemon rind, and black pepper in a paper bag. Shake well to mix, and set aside. Preheat oven to

400 degrees. Spray a 9×13-inch baking sheet with nonstick cooking spray, then coat with canola oil. Rinse cod and lightly sprinkle salt (optional) on both sides of the fillets. Cut fish into long strips. In a small bowl, combine the egg whites and milk, and whisk with a fork until well blended. Dip the fish into the egg-and-milk mixture. Place the fish strips, a few at a time, into the paper bag. Hold the bag closed, and shake well. Place the coated fish sticks on the baking sheet. Bake until golden brown, about 15 minutes.

Fish switch: You can use catfish or flounder in place of the cod.

Nutrition information per serving: 256 calories, 7.5 g fat, 2 g saturated fat, 58 mg cholesterol, 350 mg sodium, 20.5 g carbohydrate, 1 g dietary fiber, 25 g protein.

. . . .

Pronto Pasta
. . . .

Makes 4 servings

Ingredients:

1 8-ounce package whole wheat pasta

1 tablespoon olive oil

1 teaspoon garlic, minced

4 cups assorted vegetables, cut in small pieces (such as broccoli florets, sliced carrots, sliced zucchini)

1 5.5-ounce can low-sodium, diced tomatoes

1 5.5-ounce can low-sodium tomato sauce

¼ teaspoon black pepper

¼ cup low-fat grated parmesan cheese

Directions:

Cook pasta according to package directions. While the pasta is cooking, combine oil and garlic in a skillet and cook about 30 seconds over medium heat. Add vegetables and cook until they are tender, stirring occasionally. Add diced tomatoes, tomato sauce, and black pepper. Bring to a boil. Reduce heat and simmer for 5 minutes. Add pasta and parmesan cheese to the vegetable mixture. Toss until the pasta is well mixed. Serve cold or hot.

Nutrition information per serving: 359 calories, 6.4 g fat, 1.6 g saturated fat, 220 mg sodium, 66 g carbohydrate, 14.8 g dietary fiber, 16 g protein.

Quick Quesadillas

Makes 4 servings

Ingredients:

4 whole wheat tortillas (8 inches in diameter)

¾ cup shredded, low-fat cheddar cheese

1 cup diced green peppers

1 cup cooked black beans (or use no-salt-added, canned beans), drained and rinsed

Salsa (optional)

Directions:

Top each tortilla with one-fourth of the cheese, peppers, and beans. Fold tortillas in half and place on a microwave-safe dish. Microwave on high for 30 seconds or until the cheese melts. Cut each quesadilla in half. Add salsa (optional).

> *Nutrition information per serving (excluding salsa):* 250 calories, 4 g fat, 1.7 g saturated fat, 4.4 mg cholesterol, 450 mg sodium, 39 g carbohydrate, 8.3 g dietary fiber, 15 g protein.

Sloppy Garden Joes

Makes 4 servings

Ingredients:

1 teaspoon vegetable oil

1 onion, chopped

1 carrot, chopped

½ green pepper, chopped

1 pound lean ground turkey (or extra-lean ground beef)

1 8-ounce can low-sodium tomato sauce

1 15-ounce can no-salt-added whole tomatoes, crushed

1 8-ounce can mushrooms

¼ cup reduced-sodium barbeque sauce

Pepper to taste

Directions:

Lightly coat a saucepan with oil and heat over medium-high heat. Add onion, carrot, green pepper, and ground turkey or ground beef, and sauté ninutes. Add tomato sauce, crushed tomatoes, mushrooms, bar-beque sauce, and pepper and bring to a boil. Reduce heat and simmer 10 minutes, stirring occasionally. Uncover and cook for an additional 3 minutes or until thick. Serve on toasted whole wheat buns or whole wheat bread.

Nutrition information per serving (excluding bread): 240 calories, 8 g fat, 2.1 g saturated fat, 71.2 mg cholesterol, 377 mg sodium, 23.9 g carbohydrate, 4.6 g dietary fiber, 19.2 g protein.

Recipe adapted from Washington State University Nutrition Education. Eat Better, Eat Together Tool Kit: Ideas for Promoting Positive Family Meals. *http://nutrition.wsu.edu.*

Speedy Stir-Fry Rice

Makes 6 servings

Ingredients:

2 cups instant white or brown rice

6 to 8 ounces frozen, precooked salad-size shrimp (optional)

Nonstick cooking spray

6 eggs, beaten

1 tablespoon vegetable oil

3 green onions, chopped

1½ cup frozen mixed vegetables, thawed

4 tablespoons reduced-sodium soy sauce

Directions:

Prepare rice according to package directions for the microwave. If using shrimp, thaw in cold water; drain well and pat dry with paper towels. Coat a wok or large skillet with the nonstick cooking spray, and heat until a drop of water sizzles. Scramble eggs in the wok or skillet, and set aside. Add the vegetable oil, green onions, vegetables, and shrimp to the wok or skillet, and stir-fry over high heat for about 5 minutes. Add the cooked rice, eggs, and soy sauce, and stir-fry for another 3 minutes.

Nutrition information per serving (excluding shrimp): 260 calories, 6.9 g fat, 1.5 g saturated fat, 180 mg cholesterol, 350 mg sodium, 35.8 g carbohydrate, 2.7 g dietary fiber, 10.6 g protein.

Spicy Southern Barbeque Chicken

Makes 6 servings

Ingredients:

3 pounds chicken parts (breasts, legs, and thighs), skin and fat removed

1 large onion, thinly sliced

3 tablespoons vinegar

3 tablespoons low-sodium Worcestershire sauce

2 tablespoons brown sugar

Black pepper to taste

1 tablespoon hot pepper flakes

1 tablespoon chili powder

1 cup low-fat, reduced-sodium chicken stock or broth

Directions:

Preheat oven to 350 degrees. Place chicken in a 13×9×2-inch baking dish. Arrange onion over the top. Mix together vinegar, Worcestershire sauce, brown sugar, black pepper, hot pepper flakes, chili powder, and stock. Pour over the chicken and bake, basting occasionally, for 1 hour or until chicken is thoroughly cooked (to a minimum internal temperature of 165 degrees).

Nutrition information per serving: 199 calories, 4.2 g fat, 1.2 g saturated fat, 92.8 mg cholesterol, 304.9 mg sodium, 6.1 g carbohydrate, 0 g dietary fiber, 31.5 g protein.

Recipe adapted from National Heart, Lung, and Blood Institute. Stay Young at Heart: Cooking the Heart Healthy Way. *www.nhlbi.nih.gov/health/public /heart/other/syah/index.htm.*

Turkey Burgers

Makes 4 servings

Ingredients:

12 ounces lean ground turkey

½ cup green onions, sliced

¼ teaspoon black pepper

1 large egg, lightly beaten

Olive oil

Directions:

Preheat oven broiler on high temperature or preheat grill on medium heat. Combine turkey, green onions, black pepper, and egg, and mix well. Form into ½-inch to ¾-inch thick patties, and coat each lightly with olive oil. Broil or grill burgers for about 7 to 9 minutes on each side (to a minimum internal temperature of 160 degrees).

Topping suggestions: Tomato, spinach leaves, mushrooms, or any other vegetable of your choice.

Nutrition information per serving: 148 calories, 8 g fat, 2.2 g saturated fat, 112.2 mg cholesterol, 98.5 mg sodium, 0.9 g carbohydrate, 0.2 g dietary fiber, 16.6 g protein.

Recipe adapted from National Heart, Lung, and Blood Institute. Keep the Beat Recipes: Deliciously Healthy Family Meals. *http://hp2010.nhlbihin.net/healthyeating/default.aspx.*

Veggie Pita Pizza

Makes 2 servings

Ingredients:

2 whole wheat pitas
½ cup low-sodium tomato
  sauce
½ cup grated, low-fat cheese
  (mozzarella or American)

1 cup raw vegetables (such as
  green or red peppers, onions,
  mushrooms, or olives), sliced
  or diced

Directions:

Preheat oven or toaster oven to 350 degrees. Spread tomato sauce on one side of each pita. Sprinkle with low-fat cheese and top with vegetables. Brown in oven for about 8 minutes, until cheese is melted. Serve hot or cold.

Nutrition information per serving: 158 calories, 3 g fat, 2 g saturated fat, 6 mg cholesterol, 330 mg sodium, 26 g carbohydrate, 4 g dietary fiber, 10 g protein.

Snacks

. . . .

Berry Blast Smoothie

Makes 6 servings

Ingredients:

2 cups blueberries

2 cups raspberries

2 cups strawberries

1 cup 100% cran-raspberry
   juice

1 cup low-fat blueberry yogurt

2 cups ice

Directions:

Place all items in a blender and blend until smooth. Pour into glasses and
serve immediately.

> *Nutrition information per serving:* 100 calories, 1 g fat, 0 g saturated fat, 0 mg
> cholesterol, 20 mg sodium, 25 g carbohydrate, 6 g dietary fiber, 2 g protein.
>
> Recipe adapted from Centers for Disease Control and Prevention. Fruits
> and Veggies More Matters Web site. *http://apps.nccd.cdc.gov/dnparecipe/recipe
> search.aspx.*

. . . .

Black Bean Dip

Makes 6 servings

Ingredients:

1 16-ounce can black beans,
   drained and rinsed

2 tablespoons low-fat sour cream

⅛ teaspoon garlic powder

⅛ teaspoon chili powder

⅛ teaspoon black pepper

Directions:

Mash beans to a smooth consistency. Stir in other ingredients. Chill in
refrigerator. Serve with whole grain pita chips, whole wheat crackers,
baked tortilla chips, or raw vegetables.

> *Nutrition information per serving (for dip only):* 50 calories, 1.3 g fat, 0.4 g
> saturated fat, 1.6 mg cholesterol, 378 mg sodium, 12 g carbohydrate, 4.2 g
> dietary fiber, 3.3 g protein.

Chili Popcorn

Makes 4 servings

Ingredients:

4 cups air-popped popcorn

1 tablespoon melted margarine

1 teaspoon chili powder

Dash garlic powder

Directions:

Mix popcorn and margarine in a bowl. Mix seasonings thoroughly and sprinkle over popcorn. Mix well. Serve immediately.

Nutrition information per serving: 60 calories, 3 g fat, 0.5 g saturated fat, 0 mg cholesterol, 30 mg sodium, 7 g carbohydrate, 1 g dietary fiber, 1 g protein.

Fruit Kabobs with Fluffy Fruit Dip

Makes 6 servings

Ingredients:

1 cup fruit-flavored, low-fat yogurt

1 cup fat-free whipped topping, thawed

1 teaspoon honey

6 to 8 pineapple chunks

6 to 8 whole strawberries

1 banana, cut into ½-inch chunks

6 to 8 red or green grapes

6 wooden skewers

Directions:

In a small bowl, make dip by mixing together yogurt, whipped topping, and honey. Cover and refrigerate until needed. Thread one piece of each fruit onto a skewer. Repeat until the fruit is gone or skewers are full. Serve with dip.

Variation: Use any of your kids' favorite fruits.

Nutrition information per serving: 64 calories, 0.4 g fat, 0.2 g saturated fat, 1.9 mg cholesterol, 26 mg sodium, 16.5 g carbohydrate, 1.1 g dietary fiber, 2.5 g protein.

• •

Frozen Yogurt Fruit Cup
• •

Makes 6 servings

Ingredients:

1 banana

8 ounces plain low-fat yogurt

4 ounces frozen berries, thawed
  with juice

4 ounces crushed pineapple canned
  in natural juice, with juice

Directions:

Line 6 muffin-tin cups with paper baking cups. Dice or mash banana and place in a mixing bowl. Stir in remaining ingredients. Spoon into muffin cups and freeze at least 3 hours or until firm. Before serving, remove paper cups and let stand 10 minutes.

> *Nutrition information per serving:* 68 calories, 0.6 g fat, 0.3 g saturated fat, 2.5 mg cholesterol, 32.2 mg sodium, 2.5 g carbohydrate, 14 g dietary fiber, 2.8 g protein.

Online Resources

Ready to charge ahead and plan some more menus for your family? Here is a list of several Web sites that provide more sample menus, menu-planning ideas and strategies, and great-tasting, easy-to-prepare recipes. Have fun and enjoy healthy eating with your family!

Eat Smart, Play Hard Healthy Lifestyle!

www.fns.usda.gov/eatsmartplayhardhealthylifestyle

This site from the U.S. Department of Agriculture Food and Nutrition provides ideas and recipes for quick, easy, healthy meals including 14 Eat Smart menus and a recipe finder database.

Healthy Eating for Families:

www.HealthyEatingForFamilies.com

This site provides delicious, family-tested recipes and meal-planning tips to help you create *Healthy Eating, Healthy Weight* family meals and snacks.

Kids Eat Right:

www.kidseatright.org

Hosted by the Academy of Nutrition and Dietetics, this site offers articles, recipes, and videos to help busy families shop smart, cook healthy, and eat right. All content is provided by registered dietitians.

Meals Matter:

www.mealstmatter.org

This Web site is maintained by the Dairy Council of California and covers all phases of meal planning including calendars, recipes, shopping lists, and more.

MyPlate:

www.ChooseMyPlate.gov

This site features practical information and tips, including sample menus and food group–based recipes, to help you build a healthy diet for your family.

National Heart, Lung, and Blood Institute (NHLBI):

www.nhlbi.nih.gov/health/index.htm

NHLBI provides menu ideas and recipes, including the *Keep the Beat: Deliciously Healthy Family Meals* cookbook developed in partnership with the National Institutes of Health We Can! program.

Appendix A

Daily Calorie Requirements for Kids and Teens

Note: The estimates in this appendix are rounded to the nearest 200 calories. An individual's calorie needs may be higher or lower than these average estimates.

Defining Activity Levels

The calorie recommendations for boys and girls take into account how many calories are burned through physical activity. As a general rule, the categories are defined as follows:

- *Sedentary* = less than 30 minutes of moderate physical activity a day.
- *Moderately active* = between 30 and 60 minutes of moderate physical activity a day.
- *Active* = 60 or more minutes of moderate physical activity a day.

Daily Calorie Requirements for Boys

Age (years)	Sedentary	Moderately Active	Active
2	1,000	1,000	1,000
3	1,200	1,400	1,400
4	1,200	1,400	1,600
5	1,200	1,400	1,600
6	1,400	1,600	1,800
7	1,400	1,600	1,800
8	1,400	1,600	2,000
9	1,600	1,800	2,000
10	1,600	1,800	2,200
11	1,800	2,000	2,200
12	1,800	2,200	2,400
13	2,000	2,200	2,600
14	2,000	2,400	2,800
15	2,200	2,600	3,000
16	2,400	2,800	3,200
17	2,400	2,800	3,200
18	2,400	2,800	3,200

U.S. Department of Agriculture and U.S. Department of Health and Human Services. *Dietary Guidelines for Americans, 2010*. 7th edition. *www.cnpp.usda.gov/DietaryGuidelines.htm.*

Daily Calorie Requirements for Girls

Age (years)	Sedentary	Moderately Active	Active
2	1,000	1,000	1,000
3	1,000	1,200	1,400
4	1,200	1,400	1,400
5	1,200	1,400	1,600
6	1,200	1,400	1,600
7	1,200	1,600	1,800
8	1,400	1,600	1,800
9	1,400	1,600	1,800
10	1,400	1,800	2,000
11	1,600	1,800	2,000
12	1,600	2,000	2,200
13	1,600	2,000	2,200
14	1,800	2,000	2,400
15	1,800	2,000	2,400
16	1,800	2,000	2,400
17	1,800	2,000	2,400
18	1,800	2,000	2,400

U.S. Department of Agriculture and U.S. Department of Health and Human Services. *Dietary Guidelines for Americans, 2010.* 7th edition. *www.cnpp.usda.gov/DietaryGuidelines.htm.*

Appendix B

MyPlate Daily Eating Plans

For each food group or subgroup, the chart shows a recommended average daily servings at all calorie levels. Recommended intakes from vegetable and protein foods subgroups are per week. For more information and tools for application, go to the MyPlate Web site *(www.ChooseMyPlate.gov)*.

Daily Calorie Level

Food Group or Subgroup	1,000	1,200	1,400	1,600	1,800	2,000
Fruits	1 C	1 C	1½ C	1½ C	1½ C	2 C
Vegetables	1 C	1½ C	1½ C	2 C	2½ C	2½ C
Dark-green vegetables	½ C/wk	1 C/wk	1 C/wk	1½ C/wk	1½ C/wk	1½ C/wk
Red and orange vegetables	2½ C/wk	3 C/wk	3 C/wk	4 C/wk	5½ C/wk	5½ C/wk
Beans and peas (legumes)	½ C/wk	½ C/wk	½ C/wk	1 C/wk	1½ C/wk	1½ C/wk
Starchy vegetables	2 C/wk	3½ C/wk	3½ C/wk	4 C/wk	5 C/wk	5 C/wk
Other vegetables	1½ C/wk	2½ C/wk	2½ C/wk	3½ C/wk	4 C/wk	4 C/wk
Grains	3 oz-eq	4 oz-eq	5 oz-eq	5 oz-eq	6 oz-eq	6 oz-eq
Whole grains	1½ oz-eq	2 oz-eq	2½ oz-eq	3 oz-eq	3 oz-eq	3 oz-eq
Enriched grains	1½ oz-eq	2 oz-eq	2½ oz-eq	2 oz-eq	3 oz-eq	3 oz-eq
Protein foods	2 oz-eq	3 oz-eq	4 oz-eq	5 oz-eq	5 oz-eq	5½ oz-eq
Seafood	3 oz/wk	5 oz/wk	6 oz/wk	8 oz/wk	8 oz/wk	8 oz/wk
Meat, poultry, eggs	10 oz/wk	14 oz/wk	19 oz/wk	24 oz/wk	24 oz/wk	26 oz/wk
Nuts, seeds, soy products	1 oz/wk	2 oz/wk	3 oz/wk	4 oz/wk	4 oz/wk	4 oz/wk
Dairy	2 C	2½ C	2½ C	3 C	3 C	3 C
Oils	15 g	17 g	17 g	22 g	24 g	27 g
Solid fats and added sugar: Maximum limit, calories (% of calories)	137 (14%)	121 (10%)	121 (9%)	121 (8%)	161 (9%)	258 (13%)

Daily Calorie Level

Food Group or Subgroup	2,200	2,400	2,600	2,800	3,000	3,200
Fruits	2 C	2 C	2 C	2½ C	2½ C	2½ C
Vegetables	3 C	3 C	3½ C	3½ C	4 C	4 C
Dark-green vegetables	2 C/wk	2 C/wk	2½ C/wk	2½ C/wk	2½ C/wk	2½ C/wk
Red and orange vegetables	6 C/wk	6 C/wk	7 C/wk	7 C/wk	7½ C/wk	7½ C/wk
Beans and peas (legumes)	2 C/wk	2 C/wk	2½ C/wk	2½ C/wk	3 C/wk	3 C/wk
Starchy vegetables	6 C/wk	6 C/wk	7 C/wk	7 C/wk	8 C/wk	8 C/wk
Other vegetables	5 C/wk	5 C/wk	5½ C/wk	5½ C/wk	7 C/wk	7 C/wk
Grains	7 oz-eq	8 oz-eq	9 oz-eq	10 oz-eq	10 oz-eq	10 oz-eq
Whole grains	3½ oz-eq	4 oz-eq	4½ oz-eq	5 oz-eq	5 oz-eq	5 oz-eq
Enriched grains	3½ oz-eq	4 oz-eq	4½ oz-eq	5 oz-eq	5 oz-eq	5 oz-eq
Protein foods	6 oz-eq	6½ oz-eq	6½ oz-eq	7 oz-eq	7 oz-eq	7 oz-eq
Seafood	9 oz/wk	10 oz/wk	10 oz/wk	11 oz/wk	11 oz/wk	11 oz/wk
Meat, poultry, eggs	29 oz/wk	31 oz/wk	31 oz/wk	34 oz/wk	34 oz/wk	34 oz/wk
Nuts, seeds, soy products	4 oz/wk	5 oz/wk	5 oz/wk	5 oz/wk	5 oz/wk	5 oz/wk
Dairy	3 C	3 C	3 C	3 C	3 C	3 C
Oils	29 g	31 g	34 g	36 g	44 g	51 g
Solid fats and added sugar: Maximum limit, calories (% of calories)	266 (12%)	330 (14%)	362 (14%)	395 (14%)	459 (15%)	596 (19%)

Abbreviations: C = cup(s); g = gram(s); oz = ounce(s); oz-eq = ounce-equivalent(s); wk = week.

U.S. Department of Agriculture and U.S. Department of Health and Human Services. *Dietary Guidelines for Americans, 2010.* 7th edition. *www.cnpp.usda.gov/DietaryGuidelines.htm.*

Index